Birth Over 35

Sheila [...]Litt, is a s[...] [...] and an advocate of home births. She [...] the [...] right to decide the place of birth and kind of care they prefer, and to make an informed choice, based on research and their own values. Women suffering post traumatic stress after birth ring her for help, and to find the confidence to deal with it. Sheila also works with mothers and babies in prison and asylum centres. An Honorary Professor of Thames Valley University, she lectures all over the world and her books are published in 23 languages.

D0276016

3 0303 0[...]8

Overcoming Common Problems Series

Selected titles

A full list of titles is available from Sheldon Press,
36 Causton Street, London SW1P 4ST and on our website at
www.sheldonpress.co.uk

Overcoming Common Problems

Birth Over 35

Second Edition

SHEILA KITZINGER

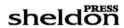
sheldon PRESS

First published in Great Britain in 1982

Sheldon Press
36 Causton Street
London SW1P 4ST
www.sheldonpress.co.uk

Revised and updated edition 1994
Second edition published 2011

Copyright © Sheila Kitzinger 1982, 2011
Illustrations copyright © Jo Nesbitt 1982

All rights reserved. No part of this book may be reproduced or
transmitted in any form or by any means, electronic or mechanical,
including photocopying, recording, or by any information storage and
retrieval system, without permission in writing from the publisher.

The author and publisher have made every effort to ensure that the
external website and email addresses included in this book are correct and
up to date at the time of going to press. The author and publisher are not
responsible for the content, quality or continuing accessibility of the sites.

British Library Cataloguing-in-Publication Data
A catalogue record for this book is available from the British Library

ISBN 978–1–84709–144–4
eBook ISBN 978–1–84709–220–5

Typeset by Fakenham Prepress Solutions, Fakenham, Norfolk NR21 8NN
First printed in Great Britain by Ashford Colour Press
Subsequently digitally printed in Great Britain

Produced on paper from sustainable forests

BLACKBURN WITH DARWEN LIBRARY	
015294222	
Bertrams	13/10/2011
618.2HEA	£9.99

Contents

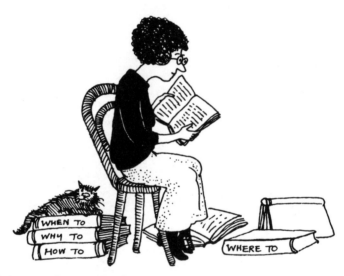

This is not a 'how-to' book

Introduction

More and more women are deciding to have a baby in their thirties or early forties. The number of 35–39-year-olds giving birth in England and Wales shot up between 1999 and 2009, and the average age was 29.4 years, the highest it has ever been.[1] Yet most books written for expectant mothers imply that they are younger, so do not give the specific information an older mother wants, or discuss the often complex emotional aspects of birth for a woman who is not merely outside the safest age range in which to have baby, but who may have a successful career, with creative and rewarding work outside the home.

This is not a 'how-to' book, packed with dos and don'ts. It is based on women's actual experiences and a wide variety of different responses to similar challenges. I am very grateful to all those who have written to me and have learned a great deal from them. Some of these were people who have been in my own childbirth classes and I was able to talk to them at length and get to know them well. The greatest proportion consisted of 289 women who got in touch following a note, requesting help, in a British national newspaper. Women in South Africa also wrote following an article in the *Johannesburg Star*, and material from 28 of their letters is included. Women sent lengthy accounts, often in astonishing detail, and were very open about their negative as well as positive reactions to pregnancy, the baby and the changes that come after the birth.

The gusto with which they wrote was expressed by one woman who, in the middle of her account, suddenly exclaimed: 'My goodness, I'm so enjoying writing all this down! It's like a confessional!' I was struck with admiration for women's courage, their capacity for giving and their strength. Many of the letters were very moving. Some were hilariously funny. The most striking thing was the generous way in which they all shared what they knew. I felt part of a great sisterhood! Sometimes there was a father's account too, or a message from older children, or from daughters who were themselves late-born children, and these were a bonus.

I had two children myself while in my thirties – the fourth and fifth in a family of five. But in this book I have concentrated on those aspects of childbirth and parenthood that women themselves talked about most often, rather than approaching it from personal preconceptions concerning what was important. The synopsis with which I started was quite different from the material that eventually emerged.

In the years since then, I have heard from hundreds of women telling me more about their experiences as older mothers.

I have not attempted to include anything about how to prepare for labour. I hope that all older mothers will seek out good childbirth classes and they may find my books helpful – among them are *The New Pregnancy and Childbirth: Choices and Challenges*[2] and *The New Experience of Childbirth*[3]. Nor is there any discussion on how to choose where to have your baby. I explore that in *Birth Your Way*[4]. I hope, however, to have written here so that a woman over 35, especially one having her first baby, and anyone having another baby after a gap, will feel she understands what is happening to her, and gains confidence to cope with the challenges before and after birth.

Sheila Kitzinger

Note: This is not a medical book and is not intended to replace advice from your doctor. Do consult your doctor if you are experiencing symptoms with which you feel you need help.

1

Deciding to have a baby

The birthdays of 30, 40 and 50 are usually presented as watersheds in a woman's life, a time for personal stocktaking, but they are also reminders of the inherent warnings of failing powers. Before the birthday in question, the woman may be seen as having potential. After it, she is often portrayed as being past her best and ageing rapidly. The cosmetic houses exploit self-doubts and fears and urge us to buy special 'youth dew'-type moisturizers and 'miracle-ingredient' creams for the 'mature' skin, 'guaranteed' to plump out degenerating cells.

This is not only a time when women may look in their mirrors more anxiously for the lines of laughter and experience, but also when they often ask, 'Who am I really?', 'What am I doing with my life?', 'Is this what I want?', and 'Where do I go from here?'

The upshot of all this is that more and more women in their late thirties and early forties are deciding that they will have a baby – either a first baby, or another one 'before it is too late', and the biological clock stops ticking.

Between 1999 and 2009 the number of 35–39-year-olds giving birth was up from 81,281 to 114,288, and women having babies after the age of 35 accounted for the greatest increase, especially in the south of England and Wales, suggesting a social-class divide. In 2009 the average age at which a woman gave birth reached a record 29.4.[1]

For others it is part of a long-term plan and what they have always intended. Some reckon to have a career and *then* babies. Though it is often believed that women having late babies must be career women who cannot make space for a child in their busy lives, research shows that only about 5 per cent of women delay motherhood for career reasons. Some women want babies from early on, but find that circumstances are against them. Claire says she would have had a baby before but could not find the right man and did not contemplate being a single mother. The potential fathers for Claire were all 'unstable divorcees' who changed their minds when it came to marriage, 'leaving me feeling deserted'. She did get pregnant 'ineptly' by 'an immature mature post-graduate', she said, but marriage did not appeal to him either, so Claire went through, in her words, 'the traumatic but fascinating experience of an abortion'. When she met a 'steady, reliable chap' a year later, they married as soon as possible and she became triumphantly, if belatedly, pregnant at 38.

A late pregnancy may occur for various very personal reasons. One is that a woman does not feel 'ready' before. As one put it: 'I wasn't mature enough to risk having a baby. I needed my work to lose my self-centredness and be aware of other people's problems. If I'd had a baby earlier I'd have been fighting for my own rights.'

Another woman delayed having a baby because everything she had read about motherhood painted a pretty depressing picture, particularly of 'non-working' mothers: 'My work was my life for 15 years. If I had given it up earlier I know I could have resented the baby.' Some women embarking on a late pregnancy even then see it as, in one woman's words, 'a hole in my career for a few years'.

Some couples have hoped for a baby for a long time, but only get down to doing anything about seeking medical help or starting the more complicated investigations and operations as a birthday crisis looms.

The over-35s are often in a second marriage or committed relationship. They may each have had children with a former partner, too. A man – especially one in his fifties – sometimes feels that he has 'done all that' and is surprised when the woman says she would like a baby. But other older men are delighted to start out on this fresh phase of their lives with the expectation of a new family. Because of such variation, this is a subject that a couple need to discuss openly, with all its implications in terms of the stresses and benefits of relationships with other children, the couple's own relationship, the financial consequences, and the extra work that a baby entails – and how it can be shared between the couple. There are probably no crystal-clear answers to the questions raised, but communicating about such matters from the start makes it much easier to cope with the inevitable challenges of parenthood by confronting them together.

It used to be thought 'high risk' to have a baby when a woman was over 30, but the more who did it the safer it proved to be. Social class and education are more important factors in safety at childbirth than a woman's age. A baby is twice as likely to die if a woman is at the bottom of the socioeconomic scale than if she is categorized as being in the 'professional' class.

The questions that weigh heavily on many older women are: 'Will the pain prove unbearable?', 'Will the baby be able to get out?', 'Am I so muscle-bound that the whole experience is going to be a terrible ordeal?' You may also hear warning bells when you go to the antenatal clinic and the obstetrician talks about you as an 'elderly primigravida'.

It is true that physiologically the best time to have a baby is in your twenties. But labour is not only a physiological event; it is also an emotional process. And the experience and understanding that an older mother may have about her body, and how to get in tune with it by way of relaxation and breathing, allows her to make better use of all the information available. She knows herself better than she did ten or fifteen years earlier too. This means she starts off at an advantage over first-time mothers in their twenties. She knows how to get on with people, how to ask questions, and to find out what she wants. This is important, for the style of birth can either be something that you passively accept or something you choose yourself. This is your pregnancy and your baby. Have it *your* way.

One of the things that most worries women over 30 is that they might have a baby with a disability and, worst of all, a learning disability. The chances of bearing a baby suffering from Down's syndrome increase slightly over the age of 30, and shoot up when a woman is past 40 (see Table 3.1 on p. 36). If you feel you would want to know if your unborn baby does have Down's syndrome, ask for amniocentesis. This is a way of detecting abnormalities in the foetus's central nervous system (spina bifida and anencephaly), and also Down's syndrome.

You are given a local anaesthetic and a hollow needle is inserted through your abdominal wall into the uterus, where about 14g of the fluid in which the baby is lying are sucked out. The baby has swallowed this fluid and passed it out of its body through its mouth or bladder. (It is full of cells from the skin and other organs that provide clues to the baby's condition.) It is then spun in a centrifuge, which separates the cells from the rest of the liquid. Since amniocentesis cannot be done until around the fifteenth week of pregnancy when some women have already felt the first fluttering of foetal movement, the decision is a distressing one to have to make and termination riskier than one performed earlier in pregnancy. A woman going through this experience needs generous emotional support from her partner.

For a woman in her twenties, the risk of having a Down's syndrome child is less than one in a thousand, so amniocentesis is a waste of time and itself introduces an extra risk, since 1 per cent of pregnancies are disturbed by the amniocentesis, causing miscarriage. For a woman of 35 to 39, the risk of Down's syndrome rises to 1 baby in every 64. This is why most obstetricians encourage amniocentesis, but not before the age of 35.

A preliminary check via a blood sample is now carried out for disorders of the central nervous system. This determines the proportion of alpha fetoprotein (AFP) in the bloodstream. If disproportionately high, this could indicate problems. Levels of AFP double about every five weeks between the fourth and six months of pregnancy, but earlier than this they are usually low. The best time to screen blood for AFP is between the sixteenth and eighteenth weeks because then it is easier to detect, the results come through in two to three days and that is usually the end of the matter.

There are two situations in which AFP may be higher than expected, but the baby is still normal: that is, if you have your dates wrong and the pregnancy is more advanced than you think, or if you are having twins (or triplets!). If there is a raised AFP level you will be offered an appointment for amniocentesis, but you may have to wait a few days. In some parts of Britain AFP testing is done on all women without telling them about it, and it can be a shock to be told that you need amniocentesis when you did not even realize that your blood was being analysed for foetal abnormalities. By this time you are aware of a living person inside your uterus and may also have had a scan and seen the baby in miniature on the screen.

With the increasing use of AFP and amniocentesis, many women feel they cannot accept the pregnancy until the foetus has been screened. One French psychologist, who studied women having babies after 40, found that it was not until they had the result (which would be four months after conception) that they allowed themselves to start looking forward to having their babies. One woman described her feelings: 'I cracked up, I burst into tears, and from that moment I was able to say – good, I must start knitting.'

To most men, and certainly to colleagues at work, the baby is not yet a reality at this stage, which makes it difficult for them to understand what a woman may be going through. For many women, if there is evidence of abnormality, there is no question but that they should have a termination and then try again, though it is a very painful decision to make if you have spent years trying to conceive.

Judy, who had already seen an ultrasound picture of her baby and had two AFP tests, both of which showed a raised level, said:

> It was the most amazing thing. What I'd thought of as a little shrimp inside me was a real baby, moving about and kicking. My baby. Now we've got to wait four days for the amniocentesis. The doctor was terribly nice about it and explained everything, but I wish they could have done it immediately. This is sheer torture!

I just don't know what to do with myself and it's as bad for John because he doesn't know how to comfort me or what to say.

It turned out that Judy was having twins!

As you get older you are more likely to have twins; the chances are highest at the age of 35, and then gradually diminish. The chance of twinning also increases as you go on having children, so that a woman in her mid-thirties who already has two or three children is the one most likely to have a multiple birth.

Having a healthy baby is not, of course, only a matter of genes, but of your whole lifestyle during pregnancy, especially in the weeks before you even know you are pregnant. In the past we have neglected those earliest weeks, treating the developing baby as if it were such a tiny speck that it could not be affected by anything we did or swallowed or breathed in. Yet more and more research is showing that the first weeks are vitally important – in many ways, more important than the later months.

I have already mentioned that perinatal mortality rates (deaths occurring after 28 weeks, at birth, or in the week following) reflect differences in social class. Improved antenatal clinics and care are unlikely to alter perinatal mortality rates until widespread social changes have improved the lives of women who are most disadvantaged, particularly those who are unsupported. Poor nutrition, smoking, industrial pollution and alcohol can kill, deform and cause learning disability in babies.

All the major organs of the baby's body are formed during the first ten weeks, and if anything goes wrong with the baby's development then, the mother cannot correct it by looking after herself better later on in the pregnancy. This is a frightening fact, especially for those near the end of pregnancy who think back to what they were doing just after they must have conceived. I am talking here about the wider-scale statistics rather than a personal recipe for damaging any particular baby. If you are not yet pregnant and plan to be, think about the environment your body provides for the developing embryo even before you conceive, making sure that you give your baby the best possible start in your uterus.

A great deal has been written about the dangers of drugs and it is true that a woman who thinks she may be pregnant should avoid all medicines unless absolutely necessary. You should be especially careful in the second half of your menstrual cycle if there is even an outside chance that you may have conceived. Most of the drugs that have adverse effects on the developing baby do most harm in the first three months.

Smoking can affect the baby's growth right through the nine months. In the earliest weeks it increases the chances of miscarriage, and after that it stunts the growth of the baby. For each cigarette smoked per day, the baby is 9g lighter and the baby of an average smoker weighs 200g less than a baby of a non-smoker. This is not so important if the baby is healthy, but it can tip the balance if it is preterm, if the mother has an illness that affects the baby's readiness to meet the challenges of life, or the mother is older than usual. Smoking reduces the oxygen-carrying capacity of the mother's red blood cells, which function 15 per cent less effectively than if she did not smoke. The lesson is clear; if you are over 30 and want to have a healthy baby, do not smoke.

Nutrition before pregnancy may be an important factor in the baby's development. One obstetrician found that when women who had previously had a baby with spina bifida were given multivitamin supplements before they became pregnant again, and for the first three months after conception, the recurrence rate of the problem was far lower than expected.

The single mother

Increasing numbers of women having babies over the age of 35 are not married. Margaret had been frightened of marriage for a long time. She had lived with a man who was violent and destructive and beat her up. When that affair finished there followed a period in which she could not trust men at all. But then she said she realized she was getting 'a bit empty inside; all those years of periods and no children'. She met a 'beautiful stranger', did not even know his surname until some months later, and could not speak his language, but knew that she passionately wanted his child. It was partly, she thinks, because she had to look after her elderly parents and their farm for many years, and partly because of an inherited puritan guilt about enjoying life, that it had all been so delayed. It was a 'one-night stand. In *Tess of the d'Urbervilles*, Hardy says that the time for loving and the man to love do not often come at the same time. But for me they did,' she says. She conceived that night.

Jane, a writer, said, 'I don't seem to have a talent for long-term and fulfilling relationships with men, but I don't see why, since I have the great good fortune to be in a position to support my own children, this should stop me being a mother.' So she had a very brief encounter with a man while on holiday on a Mediterranean island. Even so, when she discovered she was pregnant she was 'absolutely terrified' and says her mind was 'whirling round like a rat in a trap, moments of heart-stopping terror, and yet these flashes of sheer delight'. Yet another woman, in a lesbian relationship, says she felt very alone when she saw friends with their children. She was delighted to become pregnant following artificial insemination, and 'now I'm one of the pack!'

There are women living together, too, perhaps in a lesbian part-nership, who are likely to delay pregnancy until they feel sure this is the right thing to do, and that there is enough stability in their relationships for it to be the right time as well. For these, a network of loving women, rather than conventional marriage, offers a basis for embarking on the adventure of bearing and bringing up a child. Some women believe that this may be both a safer and saner environment for a child than one in which male values predominate.

A number of women over 35 who have written to me about why they got pregnant say they did so because they or their partners were unemployed or made redundant – yet one more alarming effect of an economic crisis, with long-term consequences!

'Surprise' babies

Some women conceiving at a later age are having 'surprise' babies, either totally or half accidentally. A woman concludes, for example, that she has been on the pill long enough, or that she should no longer be on it when over 35, and that it would be safer for her health to use some other method of contraception – then discovers that the alterna-tives are not so reliable. Or she comes off the pill because of its side effects and decides to 'take a chance'. Christine stopped the pill because of 'debilitating headaches':

> When I eventually realized I was pregnant no one could have been more surprised than me. My husband was shocked too, and I felt I had placed a burden on our relationship which took almost five months to untangle. I was terrified at what I had done, but as it was totally my responsibility I came to accept it.

Though she felt guilty about the pregnancy, it does take two to make a baby and maybe her husband should have been more concerned about her headaches and considered vasectomy. It is, anyway, a classic case of failure of communication between a couple. At least the crisis got them talking to each other again.

Another woman stopped the pill, had amenorrhoea (that is, her periods stopped) and was being investigated for infertility: 'I didn't know I was pregnant until I felt the baby move. At first I thought I had indigestion and had been worrying about putting on weight.'

This woman is a doctor! She wanted a baby, but realizing she was pregnant came as a great shock. A Catholic, she believes it is wrong to use any form of birth control except the 'safe period', which she admits was 'a laugh'. However, she thought it was impossible to conceive because her husband had had an operation, as a result of which he was told by the surgeons he could not father children. With five children already and very short of money, the pregnancy was a 'disaster', and she also felt acutely embarrassed to be pregnant again in her mid-forties. But she gradually came to accept 'the awful fact', and later, far from hiding the baby in the garden, as she thought she would, she 'pranced round the town showing her off'.

Jane, aged 39, mentioned above, had taken a year's leave of absence to finish writing what she calls 'a boring academic book' when she discovered she was pregnant. Her first reaction was one of panic, but when she thought about it she says that something in her was 'amazed and glad'. She was already sharing the house with a close woman friend who was excited by the news and willing to share childcare with her. Having made these arrangements, her pregnancy was 'a long, dreamy and tranquil time'. Jane felt not only special, but blessed, and she describes it as 'the St Elizabeth syndrome' (referring to Elizabeth in the Bible, who supposedly gave birth at an advanced age, having believed herself 'barren'), though other people were telling Jane that she must be mad and her own mother was 'shocked and upset', accusing her of irresponsibility. Jane found the whole experience of pregnancy and childbirth, even though it was a very painful and difficult labour, a deeply satisfying one.

Decisions, decisions

Even when conception is an accident, the decision to go ahead with the pregnancy is usually a conscious and carefully thought-out one – there is no mistake about that. Women often feel under pressure though and, like Christine, are submerged under waves of guilt. One woman said she was under pressure from her anxious psychiatrist advising her to have an abortion when she became pregnant during a serious depressive illness. She found this terribly upsetting, partly because she was feeling very pleased with herself for the first time in years. She continued with the pregnancy, feeling guilty but 'secretly rather smug' and 'one up' on the psychiatrist. By the time the baby was five months old, she no longer needed to see the psychiatrist.

Feeling guilty can mean that a pregnancy continues because the alternative seems too awful. Harriet, aged 40, went to the hospital to have a termination, where the nurse preparing her for the operation said, 'Oh dear, doctor won't like this!' Harriet got up and left. Whatever the doctor thought, it was she who was having the baby and who was committed to bringing up the child afterwards. Pressures can also be exerted the other way round and a late pregnancy be made to sound like an ominous and nasty illness, bearing such great risks of having an abnormal baby that a woman feels she cannot go through with it for this reason alone.

The single mother may have special qualms about the decision she has taken. One said that through pregnancy she kept wondering whether she was doing the right thing, but wanted it with a more consistent longing than she ever had for a man.

Occasionally a pregnancy catches the woman in her forties so much on the hop that, thinking she is beginning the menopause, she does not find out until it is too late for termination anyway. This happened in a distressing way with Elizabeth, after a brief temporary reconciliation with her former husband when she was drying out from alcoholism. One day she felt flickering movements in her abdomen and it dawned on her with horror that she was pregnant. She felt she owed it to the baby to give her up for adoption, but found it very difficult in the mother-and-baby home where most of the women, who were all much younger, intended to keep their babies. One girl told her, 'You treat it like it was throwing away dirt.'

But most women having babies at this age do so because it is what they want. And even if the decision is one that follows on the knowledge of conception, the realization brings not only shock and some apprehension, but a delighted surprise and bubbling, if submerged, excitement.

There are also, of course, second marriages, second 'chances' in life, bringing with them second, or sometimes first-off, families or at least 'one for him'. With any woman who already has grown-up or school-age children the decision-making is mixed with anxiety about how the older ones will cope. Will they see it as a loss of love? Can they handle having new family members younger than them as well as a new proxy father? What effect will a baby have on adolescents who are still very uncertain of their own sexuality and their own identity? Perhaps they will never come home; perhaps they will feel rejected and unwanted.

Some women who have babies at this age have been happy and confident in their careers and only feel able to go ahead and have a baby when they are satisfied they have achieved something in their working lives.

Rachel was 38 when she became pregnant and now has six-month-old twin boys:

> I wanted to be a person first. A wife and a mother after. I don't think women should be expected to spend their whole lives serving a man – running his home, cooking his meals, bearing his children. But I know I make a better wife and mother because I've grabbed life and done my own thing, not just slipped into the pattern Mum and Dad expected of me and that most of my friends at school fitted into without a second thought.

After getting a degree in languages, Rachel worked as a courier in a travel business, learned several more languages, spent some time in Latin America, and is now happy to be home-centred for the next ten years or so: 'Though I intend to go back into the business when the twins are at nursery school, if they can use my experience with the training courses they run.'

Motherhood in this case comes as a welcome fresh start and it is something else in which women such as Rachel hope they can also use their skills.

One woman who wrote had already decided on sterilization. Her lover mentioned having children, but she says she ignored this and assumed the remarks 'were just sentimental indulgences brought on by a new relationship'. Arrangements for the operation were delayed because the consultant was going on holiday and then had a conference to attend. During this time she began to feel having a baby with this particular partner would be a 'shared affair, and not me as a female founding a dynasty for some man'. She went ahead and had a child, though the couple did not live together and do not intend to in the future. The plan is for the baby girl to be in her mother's home for the first two months, with her father there for most of the time too, and then for the baby to move to his flat.

New responsibilities

For some women it comes as a shock that the confidence they felt in teaching or running a business, for example, wanes when faced with the responsibilities of caring for a baby, and they have to come to terms with themselves in a new way.

Delia, aged 42, had been a very capable social worker accustomed to dealing with confused adolescents, distressed mothers, those with

social problems and frail old people. She was amazed at her vulnerability and the swing of her constantly changing emotions in hospital
after having the baby: 'How could I have let them boss me around
like that? And why did I get so worked up about the changing advice
coming from all and sundry?' And when she went on feeling utterly
incompetent and dogged with anxiety throughout the first year after
the baby's arrival, she concluded that she was suffering from chronic
postnatal depression. She needed to talk about it and to be able to
get on the phone to someone supportive when she felt most isolated.
Once she was able to do this she worked through the experience, and
believed that she had learned something about herself. She is not the
invincible, all-giving person she masqueraded as. There are times when
she needs to *take* as well as to give, and she can now relax and receive
from other people as well.

Other women embark on motherhood at this age largely because
they feel they have never succeeded completely at anything else and
hope that, at last, this is something they can do. Though it might seem
they were doomed to failure and that this is one of the worst reasons
for having a baby, nearly all those who have described to me this emotional journey feel they have discovered themselves and have a new
maturity and security. Perhaps when they began to trust themselves
and had the courage to make decisions based on their own experience
of life the step was already taken, and the pregnancy confirmed this,
rather than being the cause of it.

Sue, for example, said she was a 'failed academic'. She had always
felt slightly apologetic about her job as a nursery school teacher with
her first partner, himself an academic. They were unhappy together
and the relationship broke up. Six years later she started a relationship with Dan, another academic. She gave up work outside the home
when they had a baby, and in spite of feeling diminished in status by
being 'only a mother' when she was with feminist friends who have
put mothering gladly behind them or never taken it on, she admits
that having a baby 'releases' her to 'do nothing with justification',
something she has wanted to do but has never had the confidence
to admit. One of the most important things for Sue is that she is not
alone in caring for the baby, as if it is a task only she could do and for
which innate 'maternal instincts' are sufficient. Dan shares in everything, including the night work, and is almost as involved as she is.
Because Dan does not feel it is second-class work, Sue is not defensive
about her role as a mother.

Reasons to conceive

Some babies are conceived nowadays because the woman wants satisfying work outside the home, but in the present economic situation cannot get it. Frustrated in the need for a job that meets her abilities, she opts for a baby almost as a second-best choice. This may work in the early days, but once the child is at school, she is faced with the problem again. There are added financial responsibilities and she has renewed ties at home. The baby has allowed her to bridge a difficult time, but the same difficulty reasserts itself.

One reason why a couple may put off having a baby is that one or other partner, or both, have come from an unhappy family and do not want to perpetuate this misery. One woman told me, for example, 'My own family has given me a poor pattern of personal relationships and I felt trapped in my parents' failure.' This emotional background can mean that neither partner is certain about whether it is right to have a baby. One partner usually gains in confidence through the other's love over the years, and the sense that now is the time to start out together on the adventure of parenthood grows out of the feeling of satisfaction in the couple's relationship. Without it, neither may ever feel ready for a child. Janet delayed till she was nearly 40 for this reason but is now 'hooked' on having babies. 'I am,' she said, 'like a new convert to a religion!'

Some women admit they had a baby, or another baby, for selfish reasons. 'If I had heard anyone else give this reason,' Geraldine confessed, 'I would have thought they were mad. It was quite irrational. I was very depressed, hated the house we live in, resented doing anything to it or buying anything for it.' Her three children were at school and her husband immersed in his civil service career, caught up in the 'rat race'. 'I wanted to tie myself down to the family again. I knew I was drifting away and thought I could recapture some of the happiness we had earlier in our marriage.'

Babies cannot really be used to patch a failing relationship or, at least, if they are conceived in this hope, other things have to happen between the couple before any fresh start can take place. Fortunately, Geraldine and David both responded to the challenge and, after a frightening first year or so following the birth, when she was depressed and felt she was living under a permanent black cloud, talked things through as they had never done before, and made radical adjustments in their life together. He gave up his job, which was a demanding one and meant he only really saw the children at weekends, and took another job that allowed Geraldine to do a postgraduate degree and for him to look after the family for one day a week, as well as share much more in caring for all four children. She at last feels a person again and says she has learned that 'it is too easy to become a passive dependant'. She had believed herself indispensable in this passive role, but now realizes that 'there's nothing I do for my children that they cannot either do for themselves or that someone else can do for them'. She found this to be a 'liberating knowledge' and it gives her the freedom to enjoy her children as people, rather than objects to be serviced. The stress of having a baby in an unhappy relationship can be used constructively to push the couple out of a rut, but they have to be able to make use of the experience and to *create* change, not just let things happen to them.

New dependency

For a woman who has been happily occupied with her career, however, pregnancy brings with it a new dependency in which she may luxuriate and enjoy the sense of being cherished. Sally had a demanding job in public relations and says that children were just 'things that happen to friends'. Her first marriage broke up and she remarried and started a family at 35; 'I loved being treated in a special way by everyone,' she said. This feeling of value has continued after the births of her two children largely because her husband is a 'sharing, caring partner in all things'. For other women, the sense of worth gained by the pregnancy is destroyed when caring for a new baby in social isolation. They feel drained of strength, and with it their selfhood.

Another woman who welcomed being 'taken over' by a process she trusted completely said she had had 'a great time' in her professional career, '20 years of freedom to plan my own life and spend time on what appealed to me', and now pregnancy and birth brought for the first time 'something taken out of my hands . . . to use me'. She enjoyed being in touch with her feelings in a new way, with the sense that life was expressing itself *through* her, while she learned the flexibility to respond to its demands.

Some women say that pregnancy also brings a sense of oneness with creation, even though they may never have thought of themselves as religious or mystical. The feeling of nurturing another life, of being part of a universal tradition, was how one woman described it.

Being with child also changes other people's ideas of you. 'Male colleagues at work,' one woman said, 'seem to see me in a different role. (Perhaps I'm not threatening now!) They beam at me all the time with stars in their eyes and talk about their children.' She enjoyed seeing this different reflection of self in those with whom she was in constant contact.

We do not usually put such pleasures into words, and perhaps they sound trivial when we do, but for anyone, a woman or a man, who has been scurrying around issuing documents and posting bits of paper to other people who are engrossed in the same activities, life when a baby is on the way, and being a parent, takes on a completely new meaning.

This is what happened for Shelley, who had been a cabaret dancer and an air-hostess when she married a man much older than herself and had her IUD taken out and conceived immediately. There had been no time to think about the effects on their relationship or why she was trying to get pregnant. But looking back at it now she says:

> Without doubt if Josh had not come we would have been divorced. To me, our marriage would have been like a long date and I would have packed him in as I had done with my previous boyfriends. What a blessing I hung in there because now I realize what a wonderful soulmate I have, and my happiness often frightens me.

There is another passive acceptance of pregnancy, however, which has a more negative aspect. This is the mental state in which a woman considers termination because she really does not want the child but cannot face the abortion. Ann said she was frightened and deeply shocked when she learned she was pregnant at 41. She booked an abortion, but was too confused to go through with it. For several weeks afterwards she refused to acknowledge that she was pregnant but 'when I had to accept it I was plunged into deep depression, sitting for long periods in a large armchair like a hamster in a nest'. The inner anger she felt continued, but once she started to see her doctor, and someone else obviously cared about the baby, she began to feel she could cope. In a way she handed over her emotional link with the baby. Fortunately, she and her husband could afford a nanny and she was soon back at work. Now 55, she says, 'My husband delights in her. As for me – well, I love her, but at times I wish there was no child at home.' It sounds as if both Ann and her daughter are missing out, but perhaps there is no other way.

After abortions

An older woman may have had previous abortions, and sometimes this means that her pregnancy is fraught with anxiety that she may find difficult to acknowledge. She may be afraid that she has damaged her body, or that in some way she will be punished for getting rid of an unwanted baby. For many women – probably most in fact – abortion is not an easy decision, and it casts a longlasting shadow.

In the first weeks of pregnancy a woman may relive some of the strong emotions experienced with a previous terminated pregnancy. As the months pass, she wonders what that baby would have been like, and grieves over it. The relief felt on having a successful abortion often obliterates any awareness that a woman may need to mourn her loss as well. Grieving is repressed or delayed – sometimes to emerge only much later when a woman is pregnant with a much wanted baby.

A painful longing

A woman may come off the pill when she has been on it for some years, or give up her job intending to settle down to a pregnancy at last, only to discover that she is subfertile and that it is difficult to get pregnant, or to hold on to a pregnancy that has started. Ova are less likely to ripen. After all, they have been stored inside a baby girl's ovaries since birth. They may not be released regularly as a woman approaches the menopause. Her uterus may not have the nutrients that the developing cell cluster needs in order to be implanted. There is a gradual and natural decline in fertility from the age of 28 until 35, after which the drop is steeper. When a woman is 23 her chances of having a baby are around 95 per cent. As she approaches 40, this has dropped to 75 per cent. There is a difference, however, if she is in a new sexual relationship, if only because she is likely to be having intercourse more often. It is then that her chances of success shoot up! With *in vitro* (artificial) insemination, when a woman is just past 35, six out of ten implantations are successful, at least in terms of enabling an embryo to develop for longer than six weeks. Once a woman is over 40, it is down to five out of ten.

Older women face other problems, too. They are more likely to have uterine fibroids (lumps) which, though not dangerous, make pregnancy less likely, and blocked fallopian tubes which result from infection and scarring, so that the cell cluster cannot travel along the tubes to the uterus. Women over 35 who are pregnant for the first time also have double the rate of miscarriages of women in their twenties. (If it is your second or third time round, there is no extra risk.) The chances of infertility and birth defects rise with age because of declining protein levels which act as a glue to hold chromosomes together.

There may have been a lengthy period of tests and investigations preceding a successful pregnancy. For any woman who is acutely aware that time is running out, and who desperately wants a baby, her longing becomes a painful daily reality, and the onset of each period feels almost like a miscarriage. A couple are under the continual stress of working out ovulation and the right moment for intercourse in spite of their own spontaneous feelings. The burden may become so intolerable that the relationship itself is subjected to strain. Sometimes a period is delayed just long enough for the woman to feel that this time, surely, it *must* be – but then she experiences the all too familiar sensation of the beginning of menstruation.

Susan gave up her job when she was 35, a year after she was married, to improve her chances of conception. Two years later she had a call from her doctor to tell her that her pregnancy test was positive, but she lost the baby within the next few hours. This was followed by a 'phantom' pregnancy in which she had many of the signs of being pregnant, including cessation of periods, abdominal swelling, nausea and vomiting, and what she mistakenly thought were foetal move- ments. It was a psychological trick in which her body acted out her passionate desire for a child. As a result she was very sceptical about any possible pregnancy, and when her fortieth birthday came she firmly decided that she was giving up on the idea of pregnancy and went on a 24-mile walk. She conceived the next day. She felt as if in walking the notion of having a baby out of her system she had freed her body to become pregnant.

For women who have had frequent miscarriages, or who may have experienced many years of infertility, operations, potentially dangerous drug treatments to produce superovulation, and *in vitro* fertilization, becoming pregnant in their late thirties or forties may feel like a miracle. But often it is a miracle that the pregnant woman cannot really trust. At any moment, it seems, the dream could fade, and the baby be lost. She may become very dependent upon medical advice, and rely on an obstetrician to get the baby safely delivered, rather than feel able to make her own decisions with autonomy and confidence.

She may also have come to think of her body as separate from herself, rather like a car with mechanical problems that has to have parts replaced and the engine tuned by an expert – a specialist in putting the system into running order. It is not surprising that a woman who has gone through investigations and treatment for infertility is often trapped in a medical system that is coercive and disempowering.

In traditional cultures women who do not reproduce are marked with a stigma. This is so even in our technocratic society, where they are often perceived as selfish, odd, or 'unnatural'. A woman who is pregnant after a long time of trying to conceive feels she is finally part of the human race – at last like other women. She has a sense of being drawn into a warm sisterhood with shared concerns. Mixed with anxiety about whether she can get through pregnancy and give birth to a healthy baby, there is joy that the stigma of childlessness is finally erased, and for her transformation from childless woman to 'mother'.

For many couples, getting pregnant seems to be simpler when they are on holiday and away from ordinary, day-to-day routines. Victoria and Tom were on a Greek island with other couples who had small children when they started to focus on the possibility of having more children: 'One couple there had two adorable little girls at what we call the "rubber-boot stage". ' Under the influence of relaxing sunshine and the odd bottle of retsina, Victoria said, 'Why don't we have another one or two before I'm too old?' Another couple were on vacation in Portugal where she lost her pack of contraceptive pills. They decided not to try to get hold of any more. Others were vacationing in a gypsy caravan in Spain and, during the long dark evenings when there was nothing else to do except make love, came to the conclusion that they would like to have a baby – and so made love again!

Reading all this you may feel that none of these women are like you, and that your motives are different and perhaps more complex. Whatever your situation though, it can be helpful to ask yourself, 'Why do I want this baby?' This is not because you can produce a snap answer or know exactly why, but because increased self-awareness, including understanding those aspects of ourselves that are least salutary, might enable us to be better mothers and more psychologically rounded human beings.

2

Planning ahead for pregnancy

Health is not a medical artefact. Economics, politics, the social system in which we live, conditions in the workplace, poisons in the environment, and personal relationships are all elements in causing health and disease. Doctors treat illness; they do not make us healthy.

For the vast majority of women, physical health and a sense of well-being during pregnancy is nothing to do with how often they visit the doctor, but with the social conditions in which they live – the kind of work they do, nutrition, and emotions and relationships.

Women having their first babies over 35 may have used contraception for a prolonged period, sometimes since their teens, and then make a conscious decision to stop and get pregnant. They often want to see if they can reduce stress and switch to a healthier lifestyle.

'I'm ready now'

I'd have been far too self-seeking before. I just wasn't grown-up enough to give myself to a baby and be interested in the child for his or her own sake. I would have been competing, wanting to show what a good mother I was, how I could do it better than anyone else!

Elaine had her first baby at 35 and is now enjoying life at home with three children under five:

In my early twenties I think I would have treated kids a bit like dolls to dress up and show off or like puppies to train. I couldn't have coped with crying or getting up at nights or 24 hours on duty or any of that.

Elaine didn't put off having a family for that reason, though. She was too busy doing other things. She was personal assistant to a top executive in the fashion business, and says, 'I was determined not to get sucked into the wife and home-maker thing, I wanted my own life.'

Starting a family in your mid-thirties also has advantages for children, who may benefit from having a mother who is able to enjoy them more. What some women apologize for as 'selfishness' would never be

18

seen as selfish if it was a man making the decisions. More and more women believe they have the right to decide what they want to do, to have children or not, and the right to decide at what age it is best to start a family.

The pill

Oral contraceptives have a systemic effect. Every cell in your body is affected. Artificial progesterone, on which the mini-pill – the most commonly prescribed contraceptive pill – is based, can cause masculinization of the foetus if taken during pregnancy.[1] The incidence of miscarriage and birth defects is also slightly increased.[2, 3, 4]

Oral contraceptives reduce the absorption of vitamins of the B group. When looking ahead to pregnancy make sure that you are getting a diet with plenty of these vitamins. Foods include herring and salmon, brown rice, walnuts, peanuts, wheatgerm and wholewheat products (such as bread and breakfast cereals), yeast and black molasses. Avoid liver, however, since the very high levels of Vitamin A found in liver can be toxic, and in some countries animals are still fed oestrogens to plump them up.

Pill-users also have a reduced uptake of Vitamin C. This in turn may reduce iron absorption and interfere with the synthesis of some natural hormones. The best source of Vitamin C is fresh fruit, raw vegetables and baked potatoes in their skins. A large glass of fresh orange juice every day will ensure a good basic level. All green vegetables, including parsley, broccoli and peppers, are rich in Vitamin C. One fruit source that is particularly high in this vitamin is blackcurrant.

Occasionally folic acid is low when a woman is on the pill. Alcoholic drinks reduce its absorption still further. Low levels of folic acid have been implicated as the cause of some birth defects, such as spina bifida. Include in your daily diet foods rich in folic acid: asparagus, spinach, bran, wholegrain bread and cereals, dried pulses of any kind, and yeast. Folic acid is present in liver, too, but again you may wish to avoid it. Low levels of zinc are added to cattle food. Zinc is also present in fresh vegetables, especially peas, and in wholegrain bread and cereals. Use as little cooking water as possible when preparing vegetables, or steam them. This conserves the taste better anyway. Some pill-users are also short of another trace element, magnesium. This is found in milk, nuts and wholegrain products.

Excess amounts of vitamins and minerals, especially those that are stored in the body, such as A and D, can do more harm than good. Above all, avoid Vitamin A supplements after being on the pill, since excess of this vitamin is associated with birth defects, and Vitamin A levels are raised by 30–80 per cent in women taking the pill. Levels of Vitamin A take up to three months to return to normal.[5] A nutritious balanced diet every day is the best protection against vitamin deprivation.

Though some studies have suggested that being on the pill for years reduces fertility, the great majority of women wanting to get pregnant after years on it conceive without difficulty. Perhaps those who do not had always been infertile, but did not know it. Occasionally, too, a woman in her early forties does not get pregnant because she is going through an early menopause and there are no more follicles inside her ovaries to ripen. If you come off the pill and normal periods do not return, check that you are having adequate nutrition in terms of calories. Under-nutrition reduces fertility. It is a major cause of amenorrhoea and failure to ovulate. On the other hand, some women may be slow to rid their bodies of hormones in the pill and be infertile for a year or so after. Some do not menstruate during this time. But even if you do menstruate, it does not necessarily mean that you are ovulating regularly.

If after three months off the pill you have started regular periods and notice that your breasts swell at that time, you can take it for granted that you are ovulating. If you are aware of some premenstrual tension, so much the better!

If you have had an IUD and it is removed prior to pregnancy you may possibly be anaemic, since anaemia from menstrual heavy bleeding is five times more common among women with an intra-uterine device than those using other contraceptive methods.[6] If you have a history of heavy bleeding, whether or not you have had an IUD, iron supplements may be in order before you embark on a pregnancy. Your doctor will be able to tell you this after doing a simple blood test.

Folic acid

A woman who has had a baby with a central nervous system defect – spina bifida or anencephaly – has ten times the chance of having another baby similarly affected compared with a woman whose previous baby did not suffer from this abnormality. Research in Britain[7, 8] in areas in which there is a high rate of these disabilities, with women who already had babies who suffered from these abnormalities or had pregnancies terminated because the foetus was deformed, shows that taking extra vitamins and folic acid in capsule form for three months *before* conception and during the first two or three months of pregnancy dramatically reduces the recurrence rate. All women who are planning a pregnancy should ensure that they have high levels of folic acid. If in any doubt, it is a good idea to take a 0.4mg folic acid supplement every day.

Calcium

Consider calcium supplementation, too. It approximately halves the risk of having a preterm baby and halves the risk of pre-eclampsia.[9]

Smoking

Many women who smoke stop well before they become pregnant because they know that smoking increases the risk of miscarriage, premature birth, and a small-for-dates baby as a result of a poorly functioning placenta. When a pregnant woman lights up, her baby's heartbeat speeds up, and research shows that for a smoker even to *think* about having a cigarette can have an effect on the foetal heart. The baby makes breathing movements in preparation for breathing after birth. When the mother is smoking, oxygen is reduced, these movements cease to be rhythmic, and the baby seems to be gasping. There may be long-term effects too. At the age of seven the children of women who smoked during pregnancy are slightly behind others in

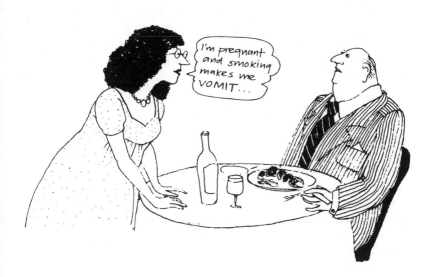

reading and some other skills. There is only one advantage to smoking in pregnancy and that is a doubtful one: a mother who smokes is less likely to develop pre-eclampsia. This is a disease peculiar to pregnancy, the symptoms of which are raised blood pressure, albumin (protein) in the urine, and fluid retention. If she *does* get it she usually has it more severely than a non-smoking mother and the outcome for the foetus is worse.[10, 11, 12]

Fathers should also stop smoking before conception. Chemical poisons in tobacco may produce abnormal sperm, and a pregnant woman should not have to breathe in a smoke-laden atmosphere – what we call 'passive smoking' – and try to avoid inhaling other people's tobacco smoke. Unfortunately it is not considered polite to ask friends, and sometimes even work colleagues, to stub out their cigarettes and it can be embarrassing when a woman is still in early pregnancy and has not yet told others about it. But some expectant mothers feel forced to do this anyway because the smell of cigarettes makes them feel nauseous. Even if you smoked before, you may be revolted by it in the first three months of pregnancy.

Though smoking reduces a baby's birth weight by 100–200g, middle-class women who smoke are fortunate in that they often have healthy-sized babies anyway. If the baby is at risk for some other reason too, and has another condition that interferes with growth *in utero*, or is the victim of poor social conditions in which the mother has to live, then that baby is most at risk from smoking. Some women who give up smoking in early pregnancy start again when they are waiting for the results of amniocentesis (see Chapter 3). They start smoking again as a result of the stress of waiting to know whether the baby is all right. If you are aware of this in advance, you may be less willing to light the first cigarette.

Alcohol

Heavy alcohol consumption is hazardous for the baby, and some women cannot safely drink any alcohol at all in pregnancy. Alcohol, even as little as one or two drinks a week, may reduce the baby's birth weight and increase the chances of miscarriage. Much of the research being done on this is retrospective, however, and there may be other factors, such as stress, poor nutrition and smoking that contribute to the poor outcome for these babies. Certainly it is known that women who smoke are also likely to drink, and those who smoke heavily are likely to drink heavily too.

In the United States the foetal alcohol syndrome is a well-known phenomenon in the babies of alcoholic mothers.[13] It is rare in the United Kingdom. These babies have learning and growth disabilities and tend to have central nervous system abnormalities and heart problems. They have a characteristic facial appearance, with a rather heavy jaw and flattened bridge of the nose.

The periods of pregnancy when alcohol most affects brain growth are weeks 12 to 18 and weeks 24 to 36. It is worth thinking this through before you become pregnant and deciding what you want to do.

Medicines

Though some drugs are known to have a teratogenic effect (producing congenital malformations) and should never be taken if you are intending to become pregnant, there are a great many others about which little is known. They may be absolutely harmless or, depending on when they are taken and the dosage, one baby in several thousand, or even 1 in 50,000 or 100,000, is affected by them. This is why it is best to avoid all drugs, even over-the-counter household medication like painkillers, if you are planning on getting pregnant. In practice, this is not always possible and it is necessary to weigh the benefits and disadvantages of taking a particular drug. Your doctor can help you with this and will have a list of medicines that manufacturers recommend should not be taken in pregnancy, or about which not enough is known to come to any firm conclusions. But if anything is to be prescribed, tell your doctor that you are thinking of starting a pregnancy. It is also wise to throw out anything in the bathroom cabinet that has been prescribed before pregnancy. If you are away from home and become ill, even if it is just a bout of holiday diarrhoea, tell the doctor that you think you may be pregnant and ask whether the prescription is safe for early pregnancy. This is one of the things that ought to be added to foreign language phrase books!

The first three months of pregnancy are those when the foetus is most vulnerable, since it is then that the main structures of the body are being formed. At two and a half months the placenta starts functioning. It is often described as a filter, but in fact it is a sieve that allows through many drugs, depending on their molecular size.

Drugs to be avoided (either because the risks outweigh the therapeutic benefits or safer alternatives are available)

- Barbiturates (sleeping pills)
- Diethylstilboestrol (DES) (synthetic oestrogen)

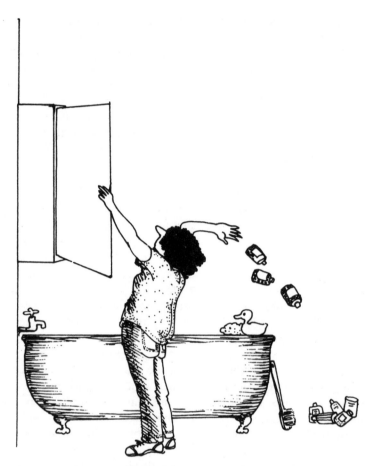

Throw out anything in the bathroom cupboard which has been prescribed before pregnancy

- Ganglion-blocking agents (to treat trigeminal neurological cyst-like enlargements on nerves)
- Iodides and iodine (anti-bacterial and anti-thyroid)
- Methotrexate (for psoriasis)
- Monoamine oxidase inhibitors (physical and mental stimulants)
- Oral hypoglycaemic agents (to decrease blood sugar)
- Oral progestogens (synthetic progesterone)
- Live viral vaccines (rubella, smallpox, tetracyclines, measles, polio and yellow fever)

Drugs best avoided

- Antacids
- Iron supplements
- Metronidazole (anti-bacterial)
- Co-trimoxaole (anti-bacterial)
- Diazoxide (to treat high blood pressure)
- Ergotamine (to treat migraine)
- Hypnotics (sleep inducing)
- Propranolol (to treat high blood pressure and anxiety)
- Prostaglandin synthetase inhibitors (to treat depression)
- Thiazide diuretics (water pills)

Drugs used under specialist supervision

- Aminoglycoside antibiotics
- Anticoagulants (to reduce blood clotting)
- Antithyroid drugs
- Cytotoxic drugs (for cancer)
- Hypotensive agents (to lower blood pressure)
- Lithium carbonate (used in mental illness)
- Systemic corticosteroids (for asthma)

Barbiturates cross the placenta rapidly, can alter the baby's fluid balance, may cause goitre and, if taken near the end of pregnancy, interfere with the baby's breathing at birth. They should be avoided in pregnancy. DES (diethylstilboestrol) is a notorious drug that can cause a special kind of cancer of the vagina in the daughters of women who have taken it at the beginning of pregnancy. It was used in an attempt to prevent miscarriages, but was ineffective anyway. Iodides are used for the treatment of thyroid conditions, cross the placenta, and can cause hyperthyroidism (overactivity of the thyroid gland) and goitre (enlargement of the gland) in the baby. Some cough medicines contain large quantities of iodides.

Live viral vaccines may infect the baby. Rubella (German measles) vaccine is of this kind. Check with your doctor that you are immune, and if you need immunizing postpone pregnancy for three months afterwards. It is also a wise precaution not to have another child in the house vaccinated against rubella if you intend to get pregnant in the near future. Monoamine oxidase inhibitors are psychotropic drugs from which a woman needs to be weaned gradually, best of all before she becomes pregnant, but if not, soon afterwards.

If you are diabetic and hoping to become pregnant, discuss this with your specialist before you conceive. Resperine, used to lower blood pressure, should not be used in pregnancy as it may slow down the heart rate of the foetus, interfere with the baby's temperature control after birth, and make him drowsy at delivery. Babies of mothers who have been on resperine may also get swelling of the mucous membrane in their noses so that they cannot breathe. Tetracycline, an antibiotic, is on the list of drugs to be avoided because it can cause a yellow stain on the baby's first teeth and slow down bone growth. The sulpha drugs, used to treat bacterial infections such as cystitis and streptococcal infections, interfere with folic acid synthesis, though they have been used for many years.

Some people think the more iron you can get, the better. This is not true, because taking iron pills unnecessarily can produce haemoglobin cells that are so large that they will not pass through the finer blood vessels in the baby, who is then deprived of some oxygen-bearing blood. The routine administration of iron supplements seems unwise and often causes nausea in the first few months, and constipation right through pregnancy. Find out if you are anaemic before taking any extra iron.

Aspirin interferes with blood clotting and may cause birth defects if taken in large doses in the first few weeks of pregnancy. Because it affects blood clotting, a large amount in the week before the baby is born could cause haemorrhaging in the newborn.

Bactrim and Septrin, used to treat urinary infections, inhibit folic acid metabolism. They should not be taken in the first weeks, and since their safety has not been proved, it is best to avoid them throughout pregnancy. Ergotamine is present in migraine medicines. It may cause the uterus to contract. Migraine can be treated with alternative drugs, and preferably with rest in a darkened room before the symptoms have time to build up.

Mogadon, a sleeping pill, is sometimes prescribed in pregnancy. It crosses the placenta and is best avoided because it affects the baby's heart rate. In fact, it dopes the baby along with the mother. Propranolol, for heart disease, also crosses the placenta and can affect the baby's heart. Sometimes it has to be used, but only for cardiac disease, not for high blood pressure. Thiazide diuretics were once very fashionable to reduce water retention, combined with strict dieting to limit weight gain in pregnancy. This is dangerous.

Several drugs are known to damage the baby's retina in high doses. One is chloroquine to treat malaria. Another is chlorpromazine used in the treatment of mental illness, but no damage has been observed with low doses. Diazepam (Valium) crosses the placenta and can cause respiratory depression in the baby, poor muscle tone and feeding problems. Librium does too. (These three drugs may have to be used occasionally, nevertheless.) Lithium carbonate crosses the placenta, can alter the foetal fluid balance, and result in goitre too.

Warfarin is an anticoagulant that crosses the placenta. If an anticoagulant is necessary earlier in pregnancy, it should be replaced by heparin four weeks before the baby is due, since it stops the baby's blood clotting. Heparin does not cross the placenta. Steroids sometimes have to be taken in pregnancy for severe asthma, but if an alternative therapy works it should be used, as there is evidence of extra risk to the baby. Local and regional anaesthetics cross the placenta too. If you must have an anaesthetic in early pregnancy let the doctor or dentist know that you think you may be pregnant.

Other risks

Most people are wary of X-rays and realize that they can be cancer-inducing. If there is any possibility that you might be pregnant, or plan to become pregnant before your next period is due, avoid X-ray of the abdomen, pelvis or lower back. The risk to the baby is highest in the first 12 weeks, and if the foetus is exposed to 25 rads or more during this time termination is advisable. Some people suggest that pelvic X-rays, if considered necessary, should only be done in the first half of a woman's menstrual cycle in case she becomes pregnant, but the ovum may be affected whether it is the first or second half. After the twelfth week of pregnancy it has been estimated that the highest risk to the baby of developing leukaemia is in the order of 1 in 500, though it is probably a good deal lower than this.

Toxoplasmosis comes from handling cat litter, so pass this chore on to someone else before you start a pregnancy, or work out a way of doing it so that there is no chance of contact. The parasite is also occasionally found in the faeces of dogs, rabbits and pet birds. A woman with primary toxoplasmosis may miscarry or her baby have birth defects of various kinds, including abnormalities of the brain and hydrocephalus. The chances are, however, that even then the baby will be all right, since eight out of ten babies of mothers with this disease have no symptoms at all.

Check that you are immune to rubella by asking your doctor to do a blood test. The risks of a woman having rubella are well known, and girls are vaccinated against rubella when at school. Women around the age of 40 will probably have had a rubella vaccine. Two or three out of every ten babies born to mothers who have rubella in the first three months of pregnancy either die, have a heart defect, or are blind or deaf. This is a chilling statistic and is why termination is offered to any woman who has the infection at the beginning of pregnancy (see Table 2.1).

Table 2.1 Risk of rubella affecting the baby[14]

Stage of pregnancy from last period	Risk of severe defect (%)
In first 4 weeks	33
5–8 weeks	25
9–12 weeks	9
13–16 weeks	4
17–30 weeks	1

Your lifestyle

It is sometimes thought that this kind of information should not be available to women because it makes them unnecessarily anxious. My own view is that I value the facts, it is my body and my baby, and if I am to understand treatment or investigations proposed I need information.

Moreover, having this kind of information affects decisions about my lifestyle, things I do every day, that are nothing to do with medical treatment, and of which the obstetrician may be unaware. Part of preparing for a baby is to think through the way I live so that I can provide the best start possible for this new human being.

Women often wonder about exercise and whether they should slow down or give up swimming, hill climbing, long walks, cycle rides or athletic activities. If you are physically fit you will have developed physiological mechanisms that allow a foetus to tolerate the circulatory and respiratory changes which occur with strenuous exercise. Your own feelings are probably the best guide to this. The changes that usually occur to cope with exercise in pregnancy are similar to those that happen during regular athletic training; there is increased cardiac output, stroke volume, heart rate and blood volume. When you are exerting yourself, placental blood flow decreases but the baby takes more oxygen from your blood. Once you have finished exercising, more blood flows through the placenta to the baby than before.

Some studies show that a sauna can be dangerous in early pregnancy if your temperature is very high and *remains* high.[15, 16] In Scandinavia, people having saunas always get into cold water (or roll in the snow)

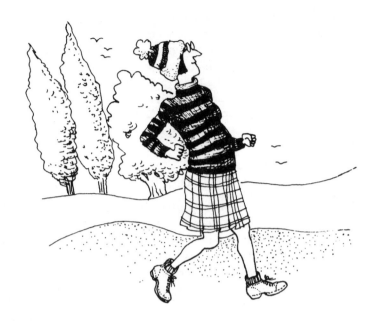

Long walks . . .

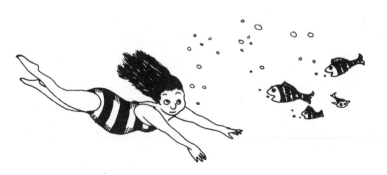

. . . swimming

afterwards. For this reason, very high temperatures, an extremely hot bath or lying under a sun lamp for a long time are best avoided. Your own comfort is probably the best guide here. If you run a high fever and think you may be pregnant it is probably better to take aspirin (see page 26) than to allow a fever to continue unabated. If the fever is not high enough to demand anything other than plenty of fluids, a cool room, and a bag of ice cubes at the back of your neck or at your temples, perhaps you can avoid aspirin. You are the best person to decide.

Diet

If you think what an Eskimo mother eats and compare this with a Masai mother's diet, both of whom bear healthy babies, you realize that no strict rules can be laid down about what you should eat, and that neither the Eskimo woman's whale blubber nor the Masai blood mixed with milk are essential items of nutrition! Most women benefit, however, from two helpings of protein each day. Be generous with fluids too, since this keeps your bladder and kidneys working well. There is no need to drink milk, though if it is only a matter of disliking it there are many ways of disguising it in other dishes. It used to be thought that liver was a near-perfect food for expectant mothers in order to prevent anaemia and give protein. But, as already hinted at, the liver and kidneys are like filters in an animal's body, and some modern methods of stock-rearing and of fattening up animals with hormone-laced feed for quick sale introduce doubts on this score. Eat wholegrain bread and brown rice rather than white. A salad as a main course each day is a good rule, with a side salad at another meal. Vegetables make a good main dish with the addition of cheese, eggs or both, or have a thick vegetable soup followed by wholewheat or rye bread with cheese. Potatoes are an excellent source of Vitamin C if cooked in their skins. A baked potato stuffed with grated cheese and herbs, with a coleslaw of finely chopped cabbage with apples and nuts, makes a good meal. Have raw fruit every day. Oranges, grapefruit and tomatoes are all rich in Vitamin C and, since this vitamin is not stored, it has to be taken regularly.

Avoid junk foods, including carbonated drinks, package mixes, bottled sauces, and most ready-prepared desserts (just look at the list of ingredients to see why). It is not a bad idea to go through the kitchen cupboards and throw out refined foods such as white flour, processed foods, and the containers you collect at the back of the shelf half full of things you never liked anyway. Bear in mind, though, that you probably have a partner who likes food too and a drastic change may be met by resistance. A new cook book that specializes in recipes for wholefoods, but without being self-consciously 'improving', may inspire both of you to experiment with dishes and stimulate your taste buds.

If your partner has not enjoyed cooking before, now is the time to begin. He needs to be able to produce nutritious and attractive meals quickly, without fuss, and to clear up afterwards. I have sometimes seen it suggested that after a baby is born women should be content to feed their families on take-aways. Yet nutrition during breastfeeding is very important if you are to feel fit, and others in the family are to enjoy their meals. Having a partner who makes good, fast food is a health plus.

It is important long before that stage, too, if you have early morning sickness and evening nausea in the first months of pregnancy. Starvation makes this worse. One way of coping is to have frequent nibbles of nutritious foods. So maybe planning for pregnancy should include a man's attendance at a course of cooking classes.

Feeling guilty

A woman may worry right through pregnancy that she has harmed her baby because she did not have the right vitamins or minerals at the beginning, enjoyed several glasses of wine at a party, had the occasional aspirin or cigarette, or because she cannot help being under stress because of money problems, or she has a violent partner.

We have already seen that a very poor diet without vegetables and wholegrains – a daily diet of hamburgers and Coke that some teenagers have, for instance – especially in the first three months of pregnancy, smoking more than five cigarettes a day throughout pregnancy, heavy indulgence in alcohol, and some drugs used to treat conditions such as epilepsy, can all cause abnormalities in the baby. But older women probably have better nutrition than very young mothers. They find greasy food gives them indigestion or heartburn when they are pregnant, so they prefer cereals and fresh vegetables and fruit. Many are guided by their own instincts to smoke less, or give up cigarettes completely. Sometimes this happens even before they know they are pregnant. If you need medication for a particular condition, your GP will be aware of which drugs are dangerous for the developing foetus, and can switch you to others that are safer.

There is a myth that once upon a time pregnant women simply budded and blossomed, and gave birth to their babies without anxiety.

Yet the evidence from women's diaries of the eighteenth and nine-teenth centuries reveals that they often worried a great deal – mainly about dying in childbirth, which in those times was a distinct pos-sibility. Women have always feared the impact of evil, unseen forces on their babies growing inside them, too. In many societies the birth of an abnormal baby is seen as punishment for wrongdoing. A curse may be set on a baby by a jealous neighbour, or the woman may see an omen in nature telling her that the baby is afflicted. Women all over the world have used prayers, charms and ritual to evade evil magic, and conformed to strict taboos, in the hope that they can keep their babies safe. In many ways pregnancy was simpler in the past. But for most of us it has never been free of anxiety.

3

Will the baby be all right?

There can be few pregnant women who have not sometimes lain awake in the darkness and wondered whether the baby would be all right. Older women, aware that the risk of congenital abnormalities rises with age, probably worry more than most.

Sometimes people believe that all the screening procedures now available can guarantee a perfect baby. Unfortunately, that is not so. There is still an element of mystery about pregnancy. In fact, this is something that many women value. Although the sperm can fuse with the ovum on a lab bench, and the cell cluster that is formed is able to grow in a glass dish, a baby needs a placenta, and to develop in a female body.

You may want the full range of investigations that are available to test whether the baby is in good health. Or you may feel under pressure to have tests that you do not really want. You have the right to make your own decisions about screening. This is so however old you are, and however 'high risk' you are rated. Every woman should have the information she needs and be able to come to her own conclusions. These may be different with different pregnancies. One woman said: 'With my first child I was prepared to go ahead with the pregnancy no matter what. This time I felt that I had to take a more responsible attitude towards my own life and well-being. I know how much work babies are this time round, and to have someone who is going to be a baby all their life seems too much to take on.' Another said, 'I had all the tests with my first pregnancy. The second time I had more confidence in myself. I knew that I could have a healthy baby. I trusted my body. So I decided against screening.'

You need not simply put yourself in the doctor's hands. You can make informed choices, valuing doctors as people with information and skills, but not handing over control to them.

Taking responsibility and making decisions

The Western medical culture of childbirth is strongly focused on the assessment and diagnosis of risk, and the pathology of birth. It is not surprising that women are often anxious and depressed as they go through a variety of tests. It has been estimated, for example, that over 10,000 women are told it is *possible* that their babies have Down's syndrome (also referred to as Trisomy 21), the most common cause of learning disability, in order to detect just one extra case.[1] Pregnancy has been turned into an obstacle course. The main weapon against giving birth to a disabled child is routine and systematic screening of all foetuses, with termination of pregnancy when the chances are high that a baby will be disabled.

When you consider the benefits and hazards of different tests, you need realistic information so that you can weigh the facts and assess risks. You will want to think about the emotional costs of screening, and the values that are important to you personally. Counselling should be readily available where screening is done, both before and after the tests, but in practice it is often only after a woman has positive test results that she has the opportunity to talk with a counsellor.

You may be certain that you want all available tests so that you can terminate the pregnancy if the baby has an abnormality, and that even tests that involve some risk of miscarriage are worth having when weighed against the possibility of an imperfect baby. Or the opposite – you are committed to having your baby whether or not there is a disability, and however severe that disability turns out to be. You may feel that you could never agree to a termination. On the other hand, like many women, you may veer between feeling that you would be silly to refuse the offer of tests, with all that they imply, and feeling protective about your baby and concerned not to get stuck on a medical conveyor belt of screening and intervention.

Probably most of us are not absolutely sure about these issues. Whatever we decide to do, it almost invariably involves other people close to us, too. Their ideas and feelings about what is right may conflict directly with our own beliefs and emotions. Taking responsibility is not simple. People are quick to comment in a critical way and, if things go wrong, blame you when your choice is not the one they would have made. There are times when you feel apologetic, defensive, guilty or angry.

Medical scientists are eager to penetrate the barriers that separate them from the 'patient' inside the uterus – your baby. Kypros Nicolaides, a specialist in this work, says, 'The barrier between the foetus and the obstetrician is being shattered. We now have access to the foetus, and the philosophy of the foetus as patient is emerging.' That barrier is, of course, the woman.[2] Tests are now being developed, and brilliant medical careers built around research that enables doctors to diagnose conditions in the foetus that were previously undetectable or only suspected. These conditions can rarely be treated at present. A diagnosis may sometimes lead doctors to reduce the length of pregnancy by induction of labour before term, to decide on Caesarean section, or in a few large centres to operate on the baby or give a blood transfusion *in utero*. But screening is not a cure. It usually raises only one question – should this baby be aborted or not?

As more and more knowledge about the foetal condition is acquired, in the future there is another question that has to be answered too. Like the first, it cannot be answered by doctors alone. What level of disability is to be reckoned too severe for a baby to be allowed to survive?

Out of 10,000 boys, 13 have an extra chromosome in every cell. It is called Klinefelter's syndrome. These boys will grow to be very tall, with arms rather larger than usual, and big hands. Some 77 per cent of them (compared with 18 per cent of all boys) have some learning difficulties, especially in reading, and just under half need speech therapy. Yet 2 of a group of 19 Klinefelter boys who were studied into adulthood have university degrees. They are gentle and sensitive, and will be infertile. If genetic tests had not been done, then most people would be completely unaware that these boys were in any way different. Would you have a termination?[3]

Many, perhaps most, seriously disabled babies would die shortly after birth if no medical effort were made to save them. In hospitals in the Western world today, these babies regularly survive, often severely disabled. Dedicated medical and nursing staff are sometimes reluctant to question the urge to treat them with all the sophisticated modern technology at their disposal. In the past the vast majority would have died within a few days. Now the many who are saved may be subjected to a great deal of surgery. As they grow older the only place that can cater for their needs may be an institution.

I do not know the answer to the questions I have raised. Perhaps there is no single answer, only the one that is right for you. But these are the issues that every pregnant woman has to face today.

Down's syndrome

Some 95 per cent of cases of Down's syndrome are age-related and result from a chromosomal disorder called a 'trisomy', when there is an extra, unpaired, chromosome. In every normal cell 46 chromosomes are arranged in 23 matching pairs. But in Down's syndrome there is an extra chromosome in the 21st pair. Another name for Down's syndrome is Trisomy 21. This is the most common cause of learning disability. Down's syndrome children have learning difficulties and may also have physical problems. As adults, they often have a happy social life, and in a protected environment can look after themselves, but remain at the intellectual level of a seven- or eight-year-old.

It is estimated that about half of all babies with Down's syndrome are miscarried early in pregnancy. Though the overall incidence of having a baby with Down's syndrome is 1 in 650 live births, the chances are low while you are still in your twenties, but start creeping up after the age of 35 (see Table 3.1).

Table 3.1 Incidence of Down's syndrome

Mother's age	Approx. risk of affected child (expressed as 1 in . . .)
20	2,000
25	1,205
30	900
35	400
36	290
37	225
38	180
39	140
40	109
41	85
42	70
43	50
44	40
45	32
46	25
47	20
48	15
49	12

If a woman has had a previous Down's syndrome baby there is a risk of 1 in 100 that another baby will be affected, unless her age-related risk is greater, in which case the risk will be higher. There are other age-related chromosome abnormalities, too, which up the chances of an affected baby (Table 3.2):

Table 3.2 All chromosome abnormalities[4]

Mother's age	Incidence (expressed as 1 in . . .)
25	527
30	476
35	204
40	73
45	23

There is a strong case for having screening – a biochemical test, ultrasound and, if indicated, amniocentesis – if you are 40 or older. Most of these tests will 'screen positive' purely because of the woman's age. This leads to terrible anxiety, even though there may be no extra risk in fact. Before the age of 40 the best action is not clear, since the investigation itself introduces a slight risk to the pregnancy. Between 1 and 2 babies in every 200 is miscarried as a result of amniocentesis. There is a greater risk of miscarriage with twins.

An older woman is more likely to have fibroids in her uterus, and the obstetrician may advise someone who is between 35 and 40 against having amniocentesis in the presence of a fibroid in case she miscarries. If you have had previous miscarriages, this also makes amniocentesis that much trickier.

Ultrasound

Most women having a baby are likely to be offered ultrasound. This consists of high-frequency sound waves, too high to be detected by our ears, which are bounced off a solid object – in this case the baby – and show up as dots tracing the shape of the baby on a screen. This is usually offered between the fifteenth and twentieth week of pregnancy, though sometimes it is suggested earlier.

Ultrasound tends to be used increasingly to take the place of information that the mother already has, and that she is perfectly capable of telling the doctor. In some hospitals there is a basic distrust of everything the patient says, and reliance is put entirely on machines. Their wholesale use for trivial reasons ('You can have a couple of scans,' one obstetrician said, 'they are rather fun') must be questioned if only because they diminish women's sense of competence and imply that the mother is a passive object of care.

A scan can confirm pregnancy from about six weeks. Besides ruling out abnormalities such as a tubal pregnancy, it reveals the foetal heart beating and foetal movements; it can also show whether you are having more than one baby. If employed in a series, a scan can be used to assess a baby's growth and, shortly before birth, the relation between the baby's head and the mother's pelvis. During the first scan a woman may be asked whether she wants to know the baby's sex, as the person operating the ultrasound may be able to distinguish this. So think in advance whether or not you want this information.

The woman is usually asked to attend with a full bladder so that her uterus is pushed upwards. She lies down, a glob of gel is squeezed on to her abdomen, and a probe on a metal arm is moved over the uterus. The whole thing takes about ten minutes. Ultrasound is used at this stage to date a pregnancy (plus or minus one week).

It is also used when biochemical tests suggest that a baby may have a neural tube defect (spina bifida or anencephaly – when the baby's brain does not grow properly). An anomaly ultrasound scan is usually done at 20 or 21 weeks. This is an especially detailed scan to investigate the baby's bones and other organs, tracking the spine for any skeletal abnormality. It can also be used to detect the skin fold at the nape of the neck as early as 11 weeks. This is called a nuchal (pronounced 'newkal') translucency scan. Babies with Down's syndrome have an extra membrane in the nape of the neck – a nuchal fold – which shows up as a black gap between the foetal neck and back. Around 85 per cent of cases of Down's syndrome babies can be discovered using this method but, like other screening procedures, it should not be considered diagnostic. The gap may show up on ultrasound and the baby still be perfectly normal. Some 3 to 4 per cent of the population have a gap of 3mm, and the majority are normal.[5] So a woman is offered chorionic villus sampling, or amniocentesis, to double-check. Ultrasound is effective in detecting severe malformation, but there is a risk of false diagnosis. In one trial 2.4 per 1,000 pregnant women were given a false diagnosis of a malformed baby.[6]

Ultrasound clinics tend to be busy, and there may be a long wait before you have a scan, and then again a wait until you collect your notes. So take something to read. One woman said:

> I was surprised that the clinic was so old-fashioned and functioned in the same way as hospitals used to years ago, with women waiting around for much longer than they should have to, doctors reading out patients' names and then marching off before they'd even made eye contact with the woman. When I had the scan there were two other people in the room, one of whom came in during the scan without introducing herself or

saying what her position was. They didn't seem to have read my notes. I had to explain I was there for dating. That was the worst bit – they didn't know why I was there. I was surprised that the hospital, which is supposed to be one of the best, was so archaic in its treatment of women.

Many women like to have their partner or a friend with them. The doctor should explain where the different parts of the baby are as they are located and measured. Practice varies in different hospitals, however. A doctor who went for her scan had to take her three-year-old with her, because her mother, also a doctor, could not get there in time to look after him, and his father, a doctor too, was at work. She was told off by the doctor doing the scan who said, 'You of all people should have known better.'

Seeing the ultrasound image

Though ultrasound is obviously a great deal safer than X-rays, it must be remembered that these were used for many years in obstetrics without anyone questioning their safety, and it was only after they were employed routinely in some consultant units to measure pelvic capacity that they were found to be carcinogenic. Tests done on ultrasound suggest that there is no hidden danger, but time may teach us differently. We can be fairly positive but not altogether sure.

Some women say that articles in magazines and TV programmes give the impression that ultrasound scans are processes in which the woman participates. They look forward to a scan as a way of learning something about the baby. Yet in some hospitals they were expected to lie down, be quiet, and do what they were told. 'My questions were either ignored or dismissed,' one said. Another woman, 'very excited at the prospect of seeing the foetus', said that the radiographer gossiped to her assistant all the way through: 'The only consolation I could draw was that she was looking at the screen and there were no sharp intakes of breath! . . . I had the feeling that a tremendous opportunity for letting the mother in on what was happening was missed.' This woman did manage to see the scan, but 'for all I know I could have been looking at a shoulder of lamb!'

It is often possible to take home a photograph of the image on the screen, but it may look more like a lace curtain with holes in it or a shifting pile of spilled pins than a baby. It can make you wonder what is growing inside you. A woman who took her ultrasound snap with her to get her blood test was 'greeted by a jolly technician who said, "Oh, you've got a photo! Can I see?" I watched as she looked at it, frowned, and handed it back with a laugh and the comment, "What I say is – you've got a fish in there!" ' This pregnant woman laughed too, but I wonder how she felt when she woke in the night, and thought about her baby.

Jan said she felt very scared at having a scan, and when she was alone with two technicians that she had never seen before she was worried that they would not know what to tell her if something was wrong: 'I didn't want to see the foetus, was very tense and felt my relationship with the baby was private.' She is one of many women who wished they had taken their partner or a friend with them.

Though some children look forward eagerly to seeing the scan, others are reluctant – sometimes for the same reasons as their mothers. They are afraid that they will bond with a baby who will never be born because it has a disability. A five-year-old boy said he did not want to see the scan, and asked his mother afterwards, 'Are you going to have the baby or not?' She was shocked by his question, because she thought it was her problem, and did not realize that it was worrying him too.

You may be disappointed not to see something that looks more like a baby. One woman said she was excited to see her baby's arm waving around. 'But it was pretty obvious it had lost its temper. It was certainly an invasion of the baby. The baby didn't like it.' Although ultrasound is not invasive of the mother in the sense that it entails sticking a needle into her or poking into her body, the shrill sound it produces (which only the foetus can hear) – and to which it reacts vigorously – certainly suggests that it is invasive for the baby.

Women often like having scans and insist on them. They make the pregnancy more real, and some start bonding with the unborn child on seeing its outline on the screen. 'It was fascinating to see the tiny arms and legs pounding away vigorously even before I could feel any movements,' said one woman. 'I couldn't have faced an abortion after that; it would have been a terrible decision!' Another woman, whose baby turned out to have serious abnormalities, commented, 'It was very upsetting that during the scan I had been shown the heart beating, and here I was two hours later being told the baby would have to go.'[7]

Yet seeing your baby on the screen as a balloon-headed, white puppet, with stick arms and legs and a spine that seems to be constructed with Lego, produces an image that often conflicts with the image that a pregnant woman has of the tiny person inside her, the seed unfolding, the soft and gently pulsing creature nestled deep in her body.

You cannot touch and stroke the image on an ultrasound screen. When the foetus reacts to the high-pitched sound with what looks like shock and pain, arms and legs shooting up, the whole body convulsed, you cannot share the baby's distress; you can give no comfort. It may be as if the baby, and your private awareness of it, has been torn from your body, as if it has become a patient to be examined – and you are left empty.

You may resist the idea that you are merely a spectator of the foetus and feel that you want to tuck the image of your baby as a real person inside your body again, and to nurture and love this child in your own way as it develops. Your knowledge about your baby, your complex feelings, all form part of what your baby is. The image on the screen is not objective reality. It is only part of the reality. The other dimensions of reality are bound up with your intimate perceptions of the baby, and with the meaning that this pregnancy holds for you. After an ultrasound you may need to reclaim your baby, and to make this child part of you again.

Alpha fetoprotein

This is a very simple blood test at 16 weeks to measure the level of alpha fetoprotein (AFP). If the level is high you may have got your dates wrong, so an ultrasound scan is done to help date the pregnancy more accurately. Or you may be having twins. The level is always high with a multiple pregnancy. Or the foetus may have an abnormality of the central nervous system. The most common kind is spina bifida, when parts of the spinal cord are imperfectly formed.

AFP is a substance that is synthesized by the baby's liver. It passes into the amniotic fluid and from there into the mother's blood. Levels double every five weeks during the middle trimester of pregnancy. High levels suggest that there may be a central nervous system abnormality. Low levels suggest that a woman is at greater risk of having a Down's syndrome baby. There is no level that clearly rules out an abnormal pregnancy. AFP concentration varies with the length of pregnancy, going steadily up until its maximum level at about 30 weeks. Between the sixteenth and eighteenth weeks the gap between normal and high levels of AFP is greatest, so this is the best time to measure it.

You may be advised to have an ultrasound scan to date your pregnancy *before* you have the AFP test. Dating is important because a high level might mean that you were further on in your pregnancy than you thought. It is also high if you are carrying more than one baby, and low if you have insulin-dependent diabetes. If the level proves to be especially high or low, you are recalled after about a week for further tests. This happens to 1 in 20 women. It is, of course, very worrying, but most women who have a high or low AFP level have normal babies. AFP testing is done routinely in some areas, and you may not know you have had it. It is worth asking. No test should ever be performed without a woman's informed consent, and without discussion of the implications of a positive result.[8]

Amniocentesis

The other common investigation is amniocentesis. This is usually done between the fifteenth and eighteenth week of pregnancy, about 14 weeks from the probable date of conception. The two extra weeks are added to date you back to the first day of your last menstrual period, which is the only date doctors think you are likely to remember accurately. Some women make up this date for convenience. If you are very unsure it is best to be honest about it, since it can affect the results of the test. Before that time there is not enough fluid. Leaving it more than two weeks would entail a more difficult abortion should you decide on termination, since chromosome culture and analysis usually take another two to three weeks. Amniocentesis can detect chromosomal abnormalities, neural tube defects such as anencephaly and spina bifida, and many errors of metabolism.

Some women hope it can ensure that they will have a perfect baby, which it cannot possibly do. A baby may have another disability than the ones that can be tested for. Ask what conditions are being screened. If you know of any disease or disability that runs in your own or your partner's family, it is a good idea to ask if screening will cover this.

You should always be able to talk through any anxieties and get all the information you need with a counsellor beforehand. One woman asked the doctor how termination would be done if this were the outcome of the amniocentesis. He dismissed her question with, 'Oh, let's not be morbid. Let's just do the amnio.' She felt put down. This particular doctor is opposed to routine screening on the grounds that it raises women's anxieties unnecessarily. But it sounds as if his own anxiety makes it difficult for him to address his patients' anxieties.

An ultrasound scan locates the pool of amniotic fluid, the placenta and the baby's position. Ultrasound is used to guide the needle into the correct space and to avoid touching the baby. Then a sample of the amniotic fluid in which the baby floats is drawn off through a needle inserted through the abdominal wall and into the uterus. This fluid contains cast-off cells from the baby which can be grown to form a culture. Results may not come for two to three weeks or longer. But geneticists now have methods of analysis that produce results in two days.

You feel a prick as the needle passes through the peritoneum covering your uterus and into the uterus itself, and the fluid is drawn off. The whole thing takes ten to twenty minutes. Occasionally it has to be done again, but not immediately because the uterus may start to contract. If you lie quietly for 15 minutes or so these contractions will fade away. Do not conclude that you have started labour.

Amniocentesis is a method of ruling out about 40 different possible abnormalities in the baby, including spina bifida, when part of the spinal column is exposed, and Down's syndrome. There is a 1 per cent risk of miscarriage – twice the risk of miscarriage in a pregnancy without amniocentesis. There is a very slight risk of infection. Some babies have breathing difficulties at birth and others have orthopaedic problems (club foot, in particular). Occasionally a false positive diagnosis results in the termination of a pregnancy with a normal baby; but this is rare.

It is important to realize before amniocentesis that it is not a question of popping in a needle like a coin in a slot and coming up with an answer. You will probably feel anxious and it is a good idea to go with a friend, especially if you know someone who has been through it before. Liz, for example, went with a friend who was two months ahead of her, 'and we were able to boost each other afterwards'. All went well, but she says it was worrying when the woman before her came out saying that they could not get enough fluid after trying four times, and she must return in two weeks. This was unusual – most units only try twice, and if unsuccessful will reschedule the procedure for another day.

'I dislike intensely the sensation of the needle going in to retrieve the fluid. The doctor made two attempts to get fluid and still couldn't get any,' Angela said. 'I would have had to go back two weeks later. I decided against it. The incident made me feel tremendously protective towards my child. The needle in my stomach felt so threatening.'

Another woman expressed her distaste of amniocentesis as an intrusion on the intimacy of her pregnancy: 'I felt the baby's privacy had been invaded with this needle going into its amniotic sac.'

Helen says that amniocentesis was 'an appalling experience', made worse because she dreaded it and knows she 'tensed up'. It wasn't helped by the lecture from the doctor on the risks of amniocentesis and being asked to sign the consent form, though this should always be done. But many women find it all far simpler than they expected. Emma said that her consultant introduced the needle very low down, after shaving off a small patch of pubic hair:

I felt a couple of tiny pin pricks and thought they were just the preliminaries. The consultant commented to the midwife that the abdomen was rather tough and he was having difficulty getting the needle through. Then I felt a niggly sensation deep inside. It suddenly dawned on me that this was the actual amniocentesis procedure itself.

You may find that the needle leaves a painful bruise, especially if another insertion had to be made. It will disappear after a few days and does not mean that any harm has come to the baby, though it is uncomfortable to have an older child climbing all over you. After amniocentesis, take it easy if you can for the next 12 hours. Sometimes when she has gone home a woman notices bleeding or leaking amniotic fluid. If this happens to you, ring the screening unit to let them know. It usually settles down without causing problems, but you will probably feel happier if you can rest in bed.

The baby's heart will be checked before you have the amniocentesis, and again afterwards, and it is comforting if you have a chance to see the baby moving on the ultrasound scan after the amniocentesis has been performed. You can ask for this if it is not suggested.

If you are rhesus negative, there is a chance of some of the baby's blood crossing the placenta, so you are given an injection to prevent the build-up of antibodies in your blood that may adversely affect the baby.

Calculating the risks

Though an older mother is at increased risk of having a baby with a chromosome abnormality such as Down's syndrome, there is no specific reason why she should be more likely to bear a child with a malformation of the central nervous system such as spina bifida.

Women having late pregnancies are often frightened of the possibility of a baby with a learning disability, particularly one with a severe condition who survives for many years. As one woman said: 'I don't know how we'd cope. It's the worst and most worrying question of all. Will our life become "lifeless" for 10, 20 years? Will we "not exist" because the child doesn't really mentally exist?' Sometimes they dread this so much that they cannot talk about it, as if, somehow, the words could create the fact.

They may dream of having a baby that is not 'right', though the mental pictures with which they disguise the image of the baby mean that they may not recognize the dream as anything related to the pregnancy. Dreams about having done sloppy work or produced an object that is imperfect and which is criticized by others (often people in authority or in uniform) seem to be one way in which a woman wraps up her fears of having an abnormal baby. These dreams, when remembered, produce a wave of distress that seems all out of proportion to the incidents that occurred. Sometimes the dream is about baby animals that are disposed of or drowned because other people decide they are not good enough or unwanted. Dreams of losing a part of your own body that has something wrong with it can also be dreams about the baby. It may be a tooth or a limb. In pregnancy, especially after you feel movement, the baby is like a part of yourself.

Knowing that disturbing and often vivid dreams are a normal part of pregnancy can be reassuring, if only because you then feel less odd. Women often do not talk about these things because they are afraid they will be upset, and perhaps even introduce ideas into other pregnant women's minds and start them worrying. In fact, a substratum of anxiety, a sense of 'What if . . .?', 'How could I cope if . . .?', is common in pregnancy, and can be a useful mental preparation for the psychological challenges that come with being a mother. None of your anxiety is being wasted. It is all grist to the mill.

Women who feel fit during pregnancy may be less nagged by doubt about the baby being normal because they know their bodies are working well. Some are vibrant with health and well-being. Many older mothers are surprised by this and describe, with delight, long walks, swimming till late on in pregnancy, enjoying sex (sometimes in a new way), and having softer skin and shinier hair than usual.

It is very different for a woman who spends much of the first three months of pregnancy with nausea and vomiting, or feeling exhausted. She asks herself whether this must not be harming the baby and is a sign that something is wrong. Her anxiety is increased, until it may become part of a spiral that is not only the result of her digestive disturbance and tiredness, but tends to increase it. When a rundown state persists after 12 weeks or so and is not cured by extra rest and sleep, it often continues until about the sixteenth week, the time when amniocentesis is performed, and disappears after. Once a woman knows that her baby is unlikely to have a congenital abnormality she can relax and enjoy her pregnancy.

It is also different for a woman who has lost a previous baby. One whose last baby had lived only for a week and who is seven months' pregnant says:

> I have either had, or imagined I had, every possible complication there is. My husband and I have only just started discussing possible names and where on earth there is going to be room for a

cot in our bulging house. A friend said to me, 'So you've finally accepted that you're pregnant', and I realized that no one apart from the children had really been allowed to talk about it.

Keeping the secret

The psychological costs of screening are often underestimated. Many women do not feel they can tell people – work colleagues and members of the family – about the coming baby until after they have had the screening results. It is as if they are not having a baby at all, in spite of the physical changes. Sometimes a woman refuses to acknowledge a baby's obvious kicking until test results have arrived because she is afraid that she will bond with an imperfect baby, whom she then must abort. To have to cope with morning sickness, or evening sickness (which is almost as common), not be able to go more than a couple of hours without a biscuit or a banana, to feel unutterably weary and drag through each day longing for bed, and then not sleep without interruption at night because of the pressure on your bladder – all while the pregnancy is hidden from family and colleagues at work – can be an intolerable burden.

If conception was accidental an older expectant mother may feel that something must be wrong with the baby. It is as if *thinking* about starting a baby makes it safer. This holds good if it means giving up smoking and having sensible nutrition before conceiving. But a happy accident need not put a baby at risk. Phyllis felt that her baby's conception had been 'freakish'. She had been working hard switching between two demanding jobs, and her husband had just got over flu. Amniocentesis set her fears to rest. A woman who already has a family may fear that this time it is not going to work out as it should: 'When you have two or three healthy children you wonder if you are pushing your luck to have another.'

When pregnant women in one area of England were asked whether they would have an abortion if it was discovered that a baby had a serious abnormality, 70 per cent said that they would continue the pregnancy.[9] In fact, if this happens the majority decide on termination. So when faced with the reality, 30 per cent of women make a decision that conflicts with their own values. The conflict, which is concealed within the concept of foetal screening, may cause anxiety, anticipatory grieving, depression and guilt. The tests a woman is offered are often seen as 'just for reassurance', but when it comes down to it, they are the first steps on a course of action that may finish with a diagnosis of abnormality and the abortion of an often much-wanted baby.

When at last it is known that the chances of the baby having a learning disability are slight and the pregnancy can be given social recognition, the whole thing becomes easier. Many women say they felt a load off their minds. One woman said, 'I felt as if a great weight had been lifted, and I realized just how worried I had been.' No test can assure you that the baby is perfect, however, though they can rule out specific abnormalities.

You may feel that there is no point in having amniocentesis if you would not want your pregnancy terminated anyway. On the other hand, you may believe that it is better to be prepared, and that knowing that the baby has a disability would help you cope better after the birth. A woman who was told that her baby had a rare form of dwarfism and would probably not survive birth decided to go ahead with the pregnancy: 'It was like living with a terminal illness. It gave me the time I needed to prepare myself for Adam's death.'[10]

It is important to think through how you feel about termination. Some women say that their doctors assumed that they would automatically have an abortion if there was an abnormality. 'It was taken for granted that a termination was necessary,' one woman said, 'I am angry that we were given no choice about it. The decision ought to have been ours alone.' Whatever decision you make, it is *yours*, not the doctor's.

Waiting for results

After amniocentesis, there follows the stressful period of waiting to get the diagnosis. Anna said this was 'horrible' and she felt in limbo. A woman who had to wait a full month commented that it was 'like waiting for exam results'. In about 1 per cent of cases a culture cannot be grown and the test either has to be done again after another couple of weeks or, if the woman is more than 20 weeks' pregnant, it may be decided to obtain a foetal blood sample, which will give a result in two or three days, or give it a miss altogether – in which case she still does not know one way or the other.

Foetal cells obtained from amniocentesis will also tell whether you are having a boy or a girl. This is only important medically if there is the possibility of a sex-linked inherited disease such as haemophilia or Duchenne's muscular dystrophy. It is usually up to you whether or not you wish to be told the sex of your baby. Some women want to keep it a surprise and believe that knowing in advance makes the pregnancy less 'normal'. Occasionally an obstetrician has a policy of never telling a woman because he does not trust her not to try and terminate the pregnancy if the baby is the 'wrong' sex. With technological power comes new responsibilities, ones that should be exercised by parents, and not only by professionals.

Chorionic villus sampling (CVS)

An alternative to amniocentesis, and one that can usually be offered earlier in pregnancy, is CVS. This diagnoses the same disabilities. A sample of tissue that forms the sac surrounding the embryo is extracted, guided by ultrasound, either through the vagina, or under local anaesthesia through a small nick made in the woman's abdomen. There is less risk of introducing infection with the abdominal route. There is a 2 per cent risk of miscarriage as a result of the test, but there is also a 2 to 3 per cent risk anyway at the stage of pregnancy when this is done – between 10 and 12 weeks.

Some 90 per cent of women go on to have successful pregnancies after amniocentesis, 86 per cent after CVS. One problem is that an apparent abnormality may be revealed that affects the placenta, but not the foetus. This may be minor. An unnecessary termination may then take place.

One woman who chose CVS said, 'It was uncomfortable, but not as much as having an IUD fitted. I lost a bit of blood afterwards – like a light period.' Her pregnancy was straightforward and the baby normal.

The advantage of CVS compared with amniocentesis is that it can be performed earlier than amniocentesis is usually done, thus enabling the woman to have a much earlier abortion if an abnormality is detected.

Complications of CVS include infection, bleeding and possibly damage to the placenta or the baby's limbs. The Medical Research Council European collaborative trial to assess the safety of this technique revealed that women who had CVS were 4.6 per cent less likely to have a live baby than those who had amniocentesis, usually because they gave birth to a very preterm baby.[11] We do not know if there are any long-term effects of CVS.

Foetal blood sampling

Another method of testing for genetic defects is foetal blood sampling, or cordocentesis. A needle, directed by ultrasound, is inserted into the baby's umbilical cord, and blood drawn off so that it can be analysed. It used to be done through the vagina but there is a risk of infection this way, and when it is done now it is usually through the abdominal wall.

This was introduced in the 1980s to test for haemophilia and other blood and metabolic disorders, immunodeficiencies (conditions in which a baby cannot resist infection) and toxoplasmosis – the disease caught from contact with cat litter or infected raw meat. Though harmless in adults, it can damage the unborn baby's nervous system.

This invasive technique has become less popular with doctors and pregnant women now that most of these disorders can be diagnosed in early pregnancy by chorionic villus sampling or, a little later, by amniocentesis.

With foetal blood sampling there is a 1 to 2 per cent rate of miscarriage. But when a woman has a 'high-risk' pregnancy – and many older women are placed in this category – the rate of miscarriage is significantly greater.

More recent techniques

Another system to assess the risk of bearing a Down's syndrome baby, one with other chromosome abnormalities, or a baby with spina bifida or anencephaly, is a form of biochemical screening called the Triple Test or Bart's Test (first developed at St Bartholomew's Hospital, London). This is a test of the mother's blood which measures three 'markers' in serum: alpha fetoprotein, unconjugated oestriol (uE) and human chorionic gonadotrophin (hCG). There is also a Triple Plus Test that uses additional biochemical markers, and that has greater accuracy. These biochemical tests are done between 13 and 23 weeks. One woman who was glad she had the Triple Plus Test said, 'They took a large amount of blood. Otherwise it was just like any other blood test. I was pleased that the results would come within a week and they would phone me directly, whether they were good or bad, rather than going through any other health care worker.'

The advantage of these blood tests is that they are followed by amniocentesis if results indicate that the chances of the baby having a disability are higher than normal. So they reduce the risk of unnecessary amniocentesis, which is a highly invasive procedure. But it is important to realize that they are not *diagnostic* tests. They cannot tell you for sure that your baby is disabled, or guarantee that it is free of disability.

If screening for abnormality is done simply by the mother's age – testing only women who are over 35, for instance – 30 per cent of Down's syndrome babies are detected. When this is combined with AFP screening, another 5 per cent are detected. But with the Triple Test, 60 per cent can be detected, and with the Triple Plus Test more than 80 per cent. The Triple Test also detects all babies who are anencephalic (when the baby's brain does not grow) and 80 per cent of those with spina bifida.

If you are thinking of having screening for abnormalities it is worth finding out exactly what tests are being offered, and their level of accuracy.

When a biochemical test reveals that the chances of a baby having Down's syndrome are 1 in 250 or more, or there is an indication that the baby could have spina bifida, the test is interpreted as 'positive'. Then it is suggested that the woman has a scan. Every test now in existence gives both false positive and false negative results.[12] False positive results often result in intense anxiety, and occasionally the abortion of a normal baby. Describing the interval between a positive result from her blood test and having amniocentesis, and then a two-week wait for results after amniocentesis, one woman said, 'They told me not to worry. But how could I not worry? It was a ghastly time. I cried a lot. I couldn't sleep. I felt drained.' Women who have had a false positive screening result may remain anxious even after they have given birth to a normal baby.[13]

By far the most usual reason for a positive screening report is that the pregnancy is not as far on as you thought. Being as little as two weeks out in your dates may change the result. Or you may be having more than one baby. Linda said:

> I didn't realize when I decided to have the Triple Test what a lottery it is – there's a chance that they'll diagnose you as probably having a Down's syndrome baby when you're not going to, and then the next step is amniocentesis which has a 1 in 200 chance of miscarriage. So you're on that route into invasive technology.

Cervical wash or aspiration

Another test for Down's syndrome is similar to a cervical smear performed to detect pre-cancerous cells. It can be done as early as the eighth week. Cells from the developing embryo are collected by washing the cervix with a sterile saline solution and drawing the fluid into a syringe. Another method is simply to suck out some cells in the cervix with a syringe. These tests are not painful and can be done in an antenatal clinic. The cells are then examined through a powerful microscope to check for abnormal chromosomes.

A termination

On the front page of the newsletter of the British organization called Support After Termination for Abnormality, there are these words: 'The decision to terminate a wanted baby because of foetal abnormality is one made out of care for the unborn child and in consideration of existing family. It is not a decision taken easily or lightly.'[14]

It may be the most difficult decision a woman ever has to make, and the pain of making that choice may bring intense suffering. It can be difficult to get any information about how termination is done and what the experience is like. One woman said, 'Nobody is willing to talk about termination till you get to the final stages of believing that there's something wrong. That's why women need midwives, not just doctors who discard our worries.' A late termination means an induced labour. Be warned that it may take 12 hours or longer. You will need a strong and loving companion with you. You may decide that it would be a good idea to make a birth plan. A woman having a termination is given a single room, but it may be on a labour ward, where others are giving birth to healthy babies, or on a gynaecology ward, where women are having social terminations and sterilizations.

When a woman has already felt her baby moving, the know-ledge that it has Down's syndrome or a central nervous system anomaly, and the decision to terminate the pregnancy, are especially distressing. Some women say that everything they do comes auto-matically and when the news is given to them it is like pressing a button to start an inevitable process for which they were mentally prepared all along. It is not so much a question of 'Why is this baby abnormal?' but 'How could I have ever thought that I could bear a normal baby?'

Your first reaction is likely to be one of shock and bewilderment. You may not be able to understand or believe what you are hearing. It seems as if it must be happening to someone else, that you must have been given another woman's results, or that the hospital has made some other awful mistake. You feel paralysed.

Some women say they reacted by feeling that if only they could go home everything would be normal again; some cannot stop crying; others freeze emotionally, and are not able to cry. The question a woman asks herself over and over again is 'Why me? Why my baby?' She usually blames herself for what has happened, and feels that if she had done something different, or avoided doing something, her baby would be normal. She may feel a failure as a woman. It may be as if she is the only person to whom this has happened, and she is trapped in utter isolation and loneliness. But there is also anger, and sometimes a desperate need to blame someone else.

It can be terribly difficult to face other people, and even to go out of the house, to talk about what you are going through with family and friends, to explain to the childbirth teacher, your mother, and perhaps your other child.

Men often feel that they must not cry and have to be strong. It can seem for a woman as if her male partner is refusing to share the grief and is just concentrating on his own life and interests. Trying to deny reality, working furiously, refusing to think or talk about the painful experience, is one way of grieving.

Most women have not revealed the pregnancy to people at work and many have not told close family members either, so they feel duty-bound to put a brave face on it and carry on as usual. They feel very alone. They often say they needed someone who understands to talk with between receiving the news and having a termination – and then again in the weeks that follow. Many hospitals provide counsellors. If you can, contact a group of women who have gone through the experience themselves. There may even be someone who can give one-to-one emotional support.

After termination

Women often say that it helped to be able to see the baby and, if they wished, to have some quiet time to hold it and say goodbye. The hospital will then help to arrange a funeral if that is what you want. You should give yourself time to grieve.

One woman said:

> It is thanks to the midwife's care and handling of us and her gentle persuasion that we were prepared to see our baby, even though at the outset this was a proposition we could not even contemplate. The midwife came back in and gently asked us if we wanted to see him. She said that if she described him it might not seem so frightening. She described him beautifully and said that she enjoyed handling him. We both knew we had to see him, thanks to her. It would after all be the last time that we three would ever be together.[15]

Suzanne was told by a doctor that at 37 she did not fall within the age group for which amniocentesis was available. 'I was strong and experienced,' she says, 'and asked if I might have an appointment with the head doctor, who readily agreed to make the arrangements.' She went back three weeks later for the results: 'I had deliberately resisted any involvement with the foetus – difficult – but I knew I would terminate if anything was grossly wrong.' The baby had Down's syndrome. Suzanne said, 'Though I had long imagined facing this news and slipped into the pattern I had prepared for myself, I was emotionally affected more than I expected. We coped with the paperwork and I asked for a quick admission.' She only had to wait 24 hours, but wonders how she would have managed without a supportive husband and doctor. The termination was efficiently and sympathetically done. She feels that someone should have told her that at this stage of pregnancy her body would react as if she had borne a live child, and that she would lactate.

After a termination for abnormality a woman may be left alone to cope. In the United Kingdom, for example, there is no statutory aftercare following a birth before 28 weeks. Home visits, concern and practical help from a midwife and doctor would be a sign that the woman's experience of pregnancy, birth and loss was acknowledged. As it is, the grieving woman is often left to get on with it as best she can; at the same time that she is bleeding, her engorged breasts are like footballs, and her whole body has to adapt to rapid puerperal change.

In the past, a woman who has delivered a dead baby would have had oestrogen pills to suppress her milk. This is no longer done because of the risk of post-partum haemorrhage (bleeding after delivery) and thrombo-embolism (a blood clot that breaks off and blocks a blood vessel). It was never particularly effective anyway, and when the oestrogen was stopped the woman often became engorged again. A better way is to bind the breasts tightly or wear a good bra, use cold compresses (ice cubes in a face towel or large handkerchief are comforting), and take analgesics if your breasts are painful. Vitamin B6 in 200mg doses has been shown to reduce engorgement for nine out of ten women. It is effective in about eleven hours and should be taken for five days.

Expressing milk encourages the supply, but on the third and fourth days, when your breasts are likely to be most hot and swollen, kneeling in a hot bath with breasts suspended in the water allows the milk to stream out without providing extra stimulation.

To have milk pouring from your breasts when you have no baby to feed is as if your whole body is weeping. For some women there is a peculiar comfort in being able to surrender their bodies completely to grief in this way. Suzanne decided not to attempt another pregnancy:

Physically I feel able to cope with termination again but it was such a difficult emotional experience I'm not certain I would want it. I had expected to value life a lot less after depriving something of life, but exactly the opposite reaction occurred.

Other women have gone on, after a breathing space and a time for grieving for the lost baby, to embark on another pregnancy, had screening again, and have given birth to normal, healthy babies with enormous gratitude and delight. They sometimes say that they did not really let the grieving go till they had had another baby: 'I didn't get the longing out of my system until Deidre was born.'

It used to be thought that a woman should wait some time after miscarriage or termination or otherwise she would be putting her next pregnancy at risk. Research now reveals that this is not so. A Scottish study shows that women who conceive within six months of losing a baby have the best outcomes and lowest rates of complications in the next pregnancy.[16] Sometimes a loving partner, anxious to protect a woman from the suffering involved, does not agree to another pregnancy. She sees this as a lack of confidence in her. It is as if he is accusing her of not being able to cope. She may resent him for treating her like a child, and feels rejected. The couple move into their separate emotional worlds.

This is what happened to Sally and Tom. She accused him of being 'insensitive' and 'cruel'. She wrote:

He was adamant that another disaster could not be allowed to occur and within three months had a vasectomy. He was totally unable to comprehend my wish for another baby which might lead to an abortion and more sorrow. We sought advice on artificial insemination but he backed out. So we are now left, often at loggerheads, and at best pushing away the fact that I still resent him.

This kind of pain can be experienced even when there are other living children. The Down's syndrome baby was Sally's twelfth child.

After she had lost the baby, one woman realized she had shut herself away from her partner's pain because it was more than she could handle, and witnessing his suffering sharpened her own ordeal. She exerted a tremendous effort of will to be cheerful because she wanted to show him and her parents that she had 'come to terms' with the experience. Tears welled up when she had locked the bathroom door, but she never allowed herself to cry in front of him. Looking back on it, she feels she made things more difficult for both of them: 'After about a week I realized he was suffering with no support from me. I'd actually forgotten I wasn't suffering alone.' Then they began to cling to each other and to share the grieving. This itself brought healing.

Following a termination for foetal abnormality a woman may feel very vulnerable and fearful. Kate said she was afraid of everything – of getting pregnant again, going on long-distance trips, flying in planes: 'I've become very fearful of death. I'm afraid I'll be punished for taking a life and that somehow I'll have to pay for it.'

It took some time for her to fully accept her thoughtfully made decision to abort her Down's syndrome baby. As her fear ebbed, she was left feeling differently about many things, especially how fragile human life is. For many months she could not face sex because of her panic at the idea of going through it all again. Then she and her partner began to reach out to each other and found comfort in sex. Now she is looking forward with excitement to another baby.

As more screening tests are devised, pregnancy is seen exclusively in terms of risk, as if it were a dangerous disease, and women become increasingly anxious. 'It is a question of whether ignorance is a blessing,' the perinatal scientist Kypros Nicolaides told me. 'We have not even begun to address the issue. I'm working at the edge of new technology, and I'm frightened of what I'm doing to women.'

4

The clinic

Understanding what goes on in the clinic is important if you are to have accurate information on which to base decisions. At the booking clinic, for which you may have the longest wait (two hours is not uncommon, so take a good book or team up with a friend) and in which tests and history-taking will be more time-consuming than at later clinics, you will be interviewed by the clinic nurse or midwife (in some hospitals by a nurse who is not a midwife). It is a good idea to discover the name of this nurse and to contact her if any worries develop or you have unanswered questions. She will ask the first day of your last menstrual period (LMP) and whether you have a regular menstrual cycle and its length. This is so that the expected date of delivery (EDD) can be worked out, by adding seven days and nine months to that day. Avoid guessing a date for the start of your period earlier than it may have been, as induction of labour may be proposed because you appear to be overdue.

She will want to know about operations and illnesses you have had, including urinary infections (such as cystitis), rubella, sexually transmitted diseases (including non-specific urethritis and thrush), and any medicines you are taking. The obstetric history includes all previous

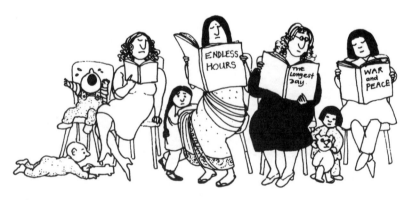

Take a good book or team up with a friend

births and abortions, whether they were spontaneous (miscarriages) or induced. Let her know if you had any pregnancy problems or birth complications before. You may also be asked questions about the health of your own family, and whether any of them suffer from high blood pressure or diabetes, and she may ask whether there are twins or triplets in the family. She will ask if you smoke and, if so, how many a day and how many alcoholic drinks you usually have. If you are not married, there may be detailed questions about housing and your plans for the future and you can also ask to have a talk with the social worker.

Someone will weigh you, as they will at subsequent clinics too, and measure your height. Though you may find the advice hectoring, if you have a body mass index (BMI) of 30 or more, it is a good idea to lose some weight *before* you get pregnant.[1] There are no evidence-based guidelines on weight gain in pregnancy. The range of possible weight gain in pregnancy is wide and there is no single 'right' or 'normal' gain. The largest weekly gains usually occur mid-pregnancy. If you gain a good deal at the start it does not mean that you will continue to put on as much weight till the end of the pregnancy. This is not the time to diet by cutting down on nutrition, though if you are gaining weight too rapidly for comfort it is a good idea to omit sugar, including the sauces, ready-prepared foods, drinks and other dishes in which there is invisible sugar. However, if you gain little weight you are more likely to have a light-weight baby than if you put on a lot; yet women who gain no weight at all have babies who are only 300–400g lighter than those who gain a great deal.

The urine specimen is another regular part of the clinic visit. It is tested for the presence of glucose (which occurs in diabetes and often, too, if you have just eaten sweet foods, such as bananas), protein (one of the signs of pre-eclampsia), and bacteria (produced by a urinary infection). You may be asked to produce a midstream sample, which is done by interrupting the stream of urine with a strong pelvic floor contraction and then letting the second flow of urine go into the container provided.

Your blood pressure will also be taken, using a sphygmomanometer. In early pregnancy blood pressure is down to lower than normal; the upper figure, the systolic, is down a little bit, but the lower one, the diastolic, is well below the non-pregnant level. During the seventh or eighth month the diastolic pressure rises to your more usual level, and under stress the upper figure, which is readily affected by strong emotion, may be high (if you are anxious or angry or have had a rush to the clinic, for example).

It may be taken for granted that you want an ultrasound scan, or a series of scans. Some obstetricians use scans routinely and tell women that they are completely harmless, although we cannot possibly know whether this is so until research into possible long-term effects has been done and accurate records kept of exposure. Unfortunately, neither of these things is happening.

At the booking clinic your heart is usually checked with a stethoscope and at the same time breasts and nipples are examined. If your nipples are inverted there is a good chance that their shape will change during pregnancy, and even if there is little alteration, once you get the baby firmly fixed on to your breast he or she will draw the nipple into the back of the mouth and mould it into the right shape. If you want to help the whole process, suggest to your partner that love play should include plenty of manual and oral stimulation of your nipples. You do not need to do anything else.

At the booking visit some blood is taken so that your haemoglobin level can be checked. If it is below ten at the twelfth week of pregnancy, you are anaemic. Your blood group is recorded in case you need a transfusion and any problems associated with being rhesus negative or ABO can be anticipated. The blood is also tested for sexually transmitted disease and antibodies to rubella. If you are rhesus negative there will be more blood tests from 28 weeks to see if you are developing antibodies. You are given an internal examination to feel the size of your uterus and the cervix and you may be offered a cervical smear to detect any pre-cancerous cells. A better time is after you have the baby.

When you are up on the couch to be examined, the doctor or midwife looks at your legs to see if you have varicose veins and, later in pregnancy, to detect any sign of swelling (oedema, a sign of fluid retention). The abdomen is palpated to see where the top of the uterus lies. The height of the fundus in relation to the pubic bone at the front of the pelvis is one way of estimating the length of gestation.

At later visits the doctor or midwife checks how the baby is lying as you get near the birth date, whether it is presenting by head or buttocks. He or she will listen to the foetal heart rate and, if you would like to hear it too, ask to do so. If Doppler ultrasound is used, you will be able to hear it anyway. This entails greasing your abdomen and passing a hand-held sonic aid over it to pick up the baby's heartbeat – you can hear this yourself with the sound turned on. It should be between 120 and 160 beats per minute – a sound like galloping horses about twice the rate of your own heart. A belt is fixed around your abdomen and the heart rate recorded for half an hour or longer. The heart is checked in this way, or using a Pinard's stethoscope, throughout pregnancy. Sometimes you are offered a continuous recording with cardiotocography (ACT).

You may also be asked to give urine over a 24-hour period to test the function of the placenta by measuring the oestriol it produces. When oestriol levels fall it is a sign that the placenta is entering its old age. A one-off specimen can give no idea at all of your oestriol levels, since output varies at different times within the 24 hours. If for any reason you are having antibiotics or corticosteroids (for severe asthma, for example), urinary oestriol levels will fall, and a low level does not mean that placental function is poor. Occasionally these tests are done on blood instead of urine. Sometimes even when results of such tests are normal, induction of labour is proposed 'because of your age'. You do not have to consent to any procedure for which you have not been given an adequate explanation.

Pre-eclampsia

Pre-eclampsia is a disease that only occurs in pregnancy. Signs are puffiness under the skin (oedema), severe headache, abdominal pain, vomiting and visual disturbances and, on examination, raised blood pressure and protein in the urine. In mild pre-eclampsia, which occurs in about 10 per cent of all pregnancies during the last few weeks, and without harming the baby, blood pressure rises to about 140/90. The lower figure is the important one as it is the resting pressure between heartbeats. In about 2 per cent of pregnancies pre-eclampsia is severe and the upper figure approaches 160, and the lower one 100, even when you are resting in bed. First-time mothers are more likely to develop pre-eclampsia than those having a second or subsequent babies. If you have had a miscarriage before, you are probably protected from pre-eclampsia, though not if you are pregnant by a new partner.

In pre-eclampsia the blood flow from the mother to the placenta is reduced.

Researchers are now convinced that though the rise in blood pressure – which is often the first sign that anything is wrong – comes in late pregnancy, pre-eclampsia is caused very early in pregnancy by damage in the tissues that later form the placenta. The hypertension (raised blood pressure) results from an imbalance between hormones that make blood vessels tighten and other hormones that make them relax. Clinical trials of supplementation with calcium, magnesium and fish oil are taking place. Some 9,000 pregnant women in 17 countries collaborated over five years with a project to discover whether a 'junior' aspirin a day helps to prevent pre-eclampsia. The idea is that the aspirin makes blood less sticky, and stops it from clotting so easily; it can then flow better. But taking aspirin in pregnancy could mean that the placenta is more likely to separate from the lining of the uterus, with the result that bleeding occurs in pregnancy, the woman bleeds too much at the time of birth, or – since the drug crosses the placenta – the baby is harmed in some way.

The baby's movements

Studies of mothers' own perceptions of their baby's movements suggest that these may be more precise than measuring the output of hormones. Any measurable changes in the placental output of oestrogen *follow* an obvious reduction in the baby's activity.[2, 3, 4, 5]

Through your awareness of movements you get to know about and be in touch with your baby in a very direct way. In the recent past, with the emphasis on modern obstetric technology, the mother's knowledge of her unborn baby's activity, its cycles of sleep and waking, and the location and nature of movements, has been largely ignored and considered irrelevant beside the 'scientific' evidence concerning placental function from urine and blood tests, ultrasound scans and other ways of getting 'windows into the womb' that are now employed. The mother has a unique opportunity, however, to get to know her baby and to be aware of movement throughout the 24 hours in a way that is impossible for any outsider. Abigail Lewis, writing of her own pregnancy, says of the foetus:

> It stretches and turns, its movements gain in power and direction. Whatever may be your own doubts about where mankind is heading and what maturity is, the foetus seems to feel no doubt at all as to what it wants; and in all that curious, segregated, seemingly static chunk of a year, you become aware of a new kind of time, the foetus's time, the slow pushing time of growth.[6]

The foetus is a water-baby in a fluid-filled capsule. Though the mother does not usually feel movements till about four and a half months, it is moving before then. Until the uterus has lifted out of the pelvic cavity into the abdomen, these movements are not felt because the wall of the uterus has no touch reception. It is only when it is lying against the abdomen that touch can be experienced. With very little gravitational pull from the earth, the baby in the uterus is like a swimmer under water, or perhaps more like an astronaut in space. Movement is easy and it twists and turns, flips from side to side and, while there is still room, before the eighth month of pregnancy may somersault. It holds on to its umbilical cord, sometimes sucks its thumb, sometimes loses the thumb and darts its head from side to side searching for it again, bounces its head against the springy pelvic floor muscles when it has dropped deep into the pelvis, presses its feet against the thick muscle forming the top of the uterus in a stepping movement, rubs its eyes with tiny fists, and sometimes the whole body jerks with hiccups.

Some of these movements may occur in response to sound. The baby hears from about the twenty-fifth week and may react strongly to loud noises and music, especially to the clash of cymbals or a brass band. At any time from about six weeks before term (the date the baby is expected) it may drop lower into the pelvis and 'engage'. If it is a snug fit, it is then difficult for the baby to make any big, whole-body movements, though it still kicks vigorously. The nature of the movements change when this happens, unless the baby is small and the mother's pelvis large, in which case it may stay equally active. The baby who is lying with its back against its mother's spine feels very active, as the limbs are at the front.

It is important to be aware that there may be a qualitative difference in foetal activity when the baby engages, in a vertex (head-down) position, facing the mother's side or back, however. If you do not know that this can happen there may be a sense of panic when the movements are more restricted. Some women notice that their babies seem to sleep for longer periods then too, rather as if the baby is settled comfortably, like the dormouse in a teapot in *Alice in Wonderland*, and does not want to be disturbed. Perhaps it is a good time for conserving energy ready for labour.

'About a week before the expected date of arrival I thought William had died because he wasn't moving,' Antonia says. 'I became absolutely hysterical. I walked down the street weeping. It took me three goes to get the nurse at the hospital to understand what I was saying, all my emotions were all over the place.' She is a single mother and she felt submerged with loneliness: 'I really needed someone to lean on then. Wow! Horrific! But the hospital said "Come up at once" and they put a monitor on the heart and he was just sleeping.'

Because women can get alarmed about not feeling movements, some doctors think it disturbing for them to be asked to note them. Some feel strongly that it is vital to reassure women at all costs and leave the worrying to professionals. Those doctors who believe this tend to favour tests that are done and analysed at the hospital, over against anything that a woman can do herself.

Yet no one would suggest that a mother should leave observation of her baby solely to paediatricians once it is born. She is the one in day-to-day contact with her child and, as such, has more intimate knowledge than anyone who sees the child only for a clinical examination. Even when she does see a professional for advice, common sense tells us that the doctor ought to spend some time finding out what the mother knows about the child and listening to her. It is purely arbitrary to say that she should do this *after* birth, but that before the baby has emerged she need not bother herself with this matter and should 'leave it to the doctors'. While the baby is still inside her, in fact, there is closer contact between the mother and her child than they are ever going to experience after the birth.

A kick chart

One good way of checking that your baby is doing well in the uterus in the final weeks of pregnancy is to keep a kick chart. It is simple to do, non-invasive and costs nothing, and can be very useful if induction is proposed since you can probably produce evidence that your baby is vigorous. A baby who is moving well when it is awake (and remember that every baby has sleeping times) is *not at risk*. It is best to pick a regular time each day when you know from experience that your baby tends to be active. Most women find that this happens in the evening when they have a chance to sit down and notice movements more readily than when they are busy and moving about. Antonia, remember, did not feel her baby move once while she was walking up and down the street. If she had gone home and got into a bath or put her feet up on the bed, she would have probably felt movements in the next hour or so.

Use squared paper, each square representing a half-hour period during your observation time. Shade in the square at which you feel the tenth movement each day. It should occur at approximately the same time, give or take 30 minutes or so, each evening.

The result will be a chart that may look something like the one in Table 4.1.

The baby in Table 4.1 is doing well!

Just before birth, the baby is likely to be a tight fit, so foetal movements are reduced, and your chart may look like the one in Table 4.2.

Table 4.1 Chart to monitor the foetus's kicking

June	Sat 1st	Sun 2nd	Mon 3rd	Tues 4th	Wed 5th	Thurs 6th	Fri 7th
5–5.30pm							
5.30–6pm							
6–6.30pm				■		■	
6.30–7pm	■		■		■		■
7–7.30pm		■					
7.30–8pm							
8–8.30pm							
8.30–9pm							
9–9.30pm							
9.30–10pm							

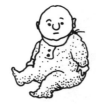

Table 4.2 Reduced foetal movements in later pregnancy

June	Sat 8th	Sun 9th	Mon 10th	Tues 11th
5–5.30pm				
5.30–6pm				
6–6.30pm	■			
6.30–7pm		■		
7–7.30pm			■	
7.30–8pm				■

If at any time you have felt no foetal movement for a full 12 hours, ring your obstetrician or the midwife at the clinic. There is no need to be alarmed, since the baby usually starts kicking soon after, but it is best to take action. One study[7] of 67 women who had no foetal movements for at least 12 hours found that 55 of them had healthy babies after a

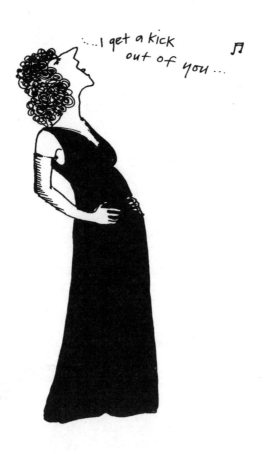

labour that started normally. The other 12 babies were passing meconium (the first contents of the bowel) or had abnormal heart rates, so labour was induced and all were born alive, ten in excellent condition and two with low Apgar rating at five minutes (the Apgar score is a system of estimating the baby's condition at birth with reference to the heart rate, breathing, muscle tone, colour and response to stimulation). If you notice a 50 per cent reduction in kicks continuing over several days, let the doctor know about it. You are your own best monitor of this, not because you are watching for danger, but because you are in touch with your own baby and know your baby better than anyone else.

If the baby is not moving the doctor may decide to do a 'stress test'. Ultrasound stimulates the foetus to move and the heart to speed up, so it is used to record reactions. If there is no response it is concluded that the baby is short of oxygen. If the baby starts kicking it is a sign that all is well. If you know that your baby usually reacts to special kinds of music, you can try the effects of this even before you go to the hospital. One woman, a singer, said her baby usually started moving when she was at a rehearsal or a concert, so she could always check how her baby was by bursting into song! If you go past your due date, your observation of the baby's kicking is even more important, as careful recording could make all the difference between labour being induced and being able to start naturally.

Your records

If you are having shared care between the hospital and your doctor you will be given a card with details of the results of examinations written in 'hieroglyphs' on it. If you are having hospital care throughout you may not get a chance to have access to your records unless you have to hold on to them while waiting in the clinic. You can ask to know what is in them and to discuss these things with the obstetricians. Though doctors sometimes think it may cause unnecessary anxiety, since the information in the records is all about the woman's body and her baby, it seems reasonable for a pregnant woman to have access to them.

Here are some of the abbreviations you may find in them:

AF	amniotic fluid
AFP	alpha fetoprotein (see page 41)
APH	antepartum haemorrhage
BP	blood pressure

BPD	biparietal diameter, head measurement. This is assessed by ultrasound, the most usual method of recording foetal growth. It is most accurate before 24 weeks, and widely inaccurate after 34 weeks. BPD grows 3.4mm a week at 17 weeks, and slows down to about a third of that at the end of pregnancy
ARM	artificial rupture of membranes
CPD	cephalo-pelvic disproportion. The baby will not go through the mother's pelvis
CS	Caesarean section
DBP	diastolic blood pressure (see page 57)
E1, 2 or 3	oestrogen output
EDD/EDC	estimated date of delivery/confinement
FBS	foetal blood sample
Fe	iron
FH/FHH	foetal heart heard
FHR	foetal heart rate
GA	general anaesthetic
GTT	glucose tolerance test, done if there is suspected diabetes
Hb	haemoglobin (see page 58)
H/T	hypertension, high blood pressure
HVS	high vaginal swab
IUCD	intrauterine contraceptive device, loop or coil
IUD	intrauterine death
IUGR	intrauterine growth retardation
IUT	intrauterine transfusion, very rare
IV	intravenous
LMP	last menstrual period
L/S	lecithin-sphingomyelin ratio, used to test maturity of foetal lungs, eg when mother has diabetes
MSU	midstream specimen of urine
NAD	nothing abnormal detected
NTD	neural tube defect
OA	occipito anterior, baby lying head down, facing mother's back. Most favourable position

OCT	oxytocin challenge test. Intravenous infusion of oxytocin while monitoring foetal heart to see how baby responds to strong contractions
OP	occipito posterior. Baby lying head down, facing mother's front. Expect long first stage of labour with backache. Keep upright and moving, if possible
OT	occipito transverse. Baby lying head down, sideways on. May move to anterior or posterior
PE	per vaginum: vaginal examination
PE2/PGE2	prostaglandin used in induction
PET	pre-eclampsia (see page 59)
POP	persistent occipito posterior
PPH	post partum haemorrhage
RE	rectal examination
SBP	systolic blood pressure (see page 59)
SVD	spontaneous vaginal delivery/spontaneous vertex delivery.
T3R	test of thyroid function
VE	vaginal examination

You will see that some abbreviations are similar to others. NAD is a very usual entry, yet it is like NTD – neural tube defect. If in any doubt about the writing, pluck up courage to ask the person who wrote it.

5

Doctors

One great advantage in being older and more experienced can be that a woman is more skilled and confident in finding out what she needs to know about the medical system, manoeuvring her way through it, and getting what she wants. This may have to start when the pregnancy is first confirmed. One woman, very happy to be pregnant by a man with whom she had lived for two years, went to a gynaecologist to make sure that all was well. He told her she was definitely pregnant and then said, 'When do you want the abortion?' 'Abortion?' she said, 'I want this baby.' 'Oh,' he replied. 'Forty and unmarried. Most unusual.' She found she had to convince the doctor that she wanted to go ahead with the pregnancy, an experience that might have thrown a younger woman.

The woman in her thirties or forties is more likely to know where to go to get accurate information, how to sift the evidence, and then negotiate the kind of birth she would like to have, in the setting of her choice.

It is easier to assume that hospital must be safer than home birth, but a review of maternity services in England found that one in five NHS Trusts put mothers and babies at risk and London hospitals were the worst. Reasons included poor antenatal care, too few staff on labour wards, and hit and miss discharge after delivery. The Chief Executive of the NHS Trust said, 'We believe that the choices mothers make about where they have babies . . . should drive patterns of maternity provision.'[1]

Despite NHS policy guidelines, out of 26,000 women in January/February 2007, 43 per cent said that they were not given the opportunity to give birth at home, and 27 per cent said that they delivered on their backs with their legs in stirrups. There were wide variations between trusts and hospitals in different parts of the UK, with Bart's and Chelsea and Westminster being the London hospitals scoring the worst.[2]

In obstetrics, as in other branches of medicine, there is a failure to confront uncertainty and it is assumed that interventions work when in fact they may introduce extra risk. Confronting this issue, an important paper on therapeutic ignorance by Iain Chalmers states that, 'Our failure to confront uncertainty about the effects of treatment has resulted in the suffering and death of patients, sometimes on a massive scale.' Formerly an obstetrician, and now co-ordinator of the James Lind Initiative in Oxford, he comments that:

> Thousands of existing questions have not yet been investigated in systematic reviews, and thousands of systematic reviews have shown that the existing evidence does not answer important questions about the effects of many treatments. This challenge will not go away – indeed, resolving one uncertainty almost always results in the recognition of additional uncertainties. The consequences for patients of acquiescing in therapeutic ignorance can be disastrous.[3]

This issue is especially important for women having babies after 35, who confront 'just in case' obstetrics and are coerced into accepting interventions 'for the sake of the baby'.

Julie was having her fourth baby at 40. The others had all been born at home and she wanted this one at home, too. She said:

> I merely told them that unless there were pressing medical contra-indications I should stay at home. One said that they might not have a midwife available. I said that didn't deter me. He said no more and a midwife duly appeared. I did need to have a certain amount of toughness.

Another woman had fully intended to have her baby in hospital, but one week before her due date visited the delivery suite to look around. She decided then and there that she was not prepared to have her baby in such surroundings, so she had a home birth.

After a four-hour wait at the clinic, Caroline was told by a junior doctor that she was to be induced. He said she would need an epidural because induced labour was always more painful and a first labour would last at least 24 hours. He told her that she must make up her mind about this immediately. When she arrived home weeping and distressed, her partner took immediate action and phoned the senior obstetrician to find out exactly what was happening, and why. Caroline was convinced by what he said – that induction was the best course of action.

The induction went well and she needed no painkillers at all. She asked for an epidural just as she was entering transition, but on learning that she was almost full dilated decided it was not necessary. 'The anaesthetist came back to give me "just a little jab to help the pain". John asked what was in this "jab" and the anaesthetist said, "Pethidine". We said "No thank you".' The baby slipped out shortly after, and Caroline was delighted to have had a spontaneous birth without any drugs. Her partner had been her ally and support in this. 'Together we had done it.' Summing up, she says, 'The process of labour and giving birth was highly satisfactory, partly I'm sure due to the fact that we asserted our rights and developed a very positive relationship with the midwife.'

In fact, for most women it is not as straightforward as that. Many say they find clinics dreadful, communication inadequate, and doctors' assumptions that patients should have a passive role leave them feeling frustrated and helpless. Carole lives in an industrial town and says everybody there has to have their babies at the infirmary. (That, in itself, is an odd name for a place to have a baby.) She had shared care and contrasts the midwives' clinic, where it is easy to discuss worries and ask questions, with the consultant clinic, where women sit or stand in long queues and 'never see the same person twice'. There are 'boxes which you wait in until you are called . . . like confessionals with a door at each end and a seat inside. The walls are bare. You cannot see another soul and it is very hot. You can be in these boxes for anything up to an hour.' In fact, she says she once sat there for two and a half hours. 'The doctor puts in an appearance, says "Good afternoon, is everything all right . . . I'll just listen to your tummy . . . Thank you, see you next week".' She never managed to extract any information about her pregnancy from the obstetrician, but nevertheless continued to attend the clinic to undergo this ritual.

Another woman, who might be considered competent in communication, since she is a post-doctoral developmental psychologist engaged in research, says that she had to 'squeeze every single piece of information' out of the doctor and was 'appalled at the whole business'. Joan refused to go to the hospital clinic after being 'treated like a moron' and had an appointment with her GP instead. Dilys, having her third baby at 40, insisted on a home birth after her experience at the clinic:

> I was handed a booklet urging me to bring any worries to the doctors. When I am ushered in to him he addresses his questions to me with his back turned while filling in my form. He turns only to look at my bulge and my vulva and never addresses any remarks to my face at all. At what point does one break in with one's inmost anxieties? Perhaps I should have gone in a frog mask just to see if he would notice?

Feeling old

Being surrounded by much younger women in the clinic can also make you feel older than you are. One woman, very conscious of her grey hairs, was told by the Sister to 'run along home, dear, we haven't time for grandmas today'. (A letter of apology arrived afterwards.) On the other hand, many women are pleasantly surprised to find that they are not alone in being older mothers and that what one woman called 'obstetric geriatrics' are becoming commonplace. Clinic staff, however, may, often inadvertently, suggest that a pregnancy and labour are going to be especially difficult. One expectant mother of 37 said that throughout her pregnancy she felt that the famous teaching hospital she attended treated her as a 'freak'.

Nancy, aged 36, said that she was trying to find out from midwives at the hospital whether she could arrange a Leboyer-style delivery and have a 48-hour discharge. They told her to speak to the senior nursing officer to find out about hospital policy. The appointment for which she asked was long delayed, so she asked the obstetrician during her next antenatal visit. He said, 'Oh, I shouldn't worry about that if I were you. At your age you are more than likely to spend the last few weeks in hospital and then to be induced or have a Caesarean.'

The woman who is having a late baby after a long gap is able to compare the present experience with previous births. If her first family are already in their late teens she spans the time during which there has been a complete medicalization of childbirth. One woman, for example, commented on the contrast between the personal care she was given when she was 20 and felt 'rather clever' at having a baby, and the impersonal, factory-farm baby production she experienced when she had another baby at 42, and remarked how 'grim' it is nowadays. Another said: 'Pregnancy and childbirth seem to be a nightmare now. People are very afraid and forever worrying about their dates and whether the baby is growing.' Several women had such bad experiences of big hospitals when they started second families in their late thirties that they insisted on having subsequent babies in a midwife-run unit or at home and were very glad they did. Some had first babies at home. They often found they had to battle for this, though occasionally it was welcomed by the doctor. Jill, aged 33, said she went to the doctor 'armed with statistics and arguments about the desirability of a home birth . . . whereupon he took all the wind out of my sails by saying, "Oh yes, that'll be rather nice. I haven't done one of those for a long time."'

The hospital doctors were a different matter. One made it clear to Jill that 'the decision about where to have my baby was nothing to do with me and would be made on my behalf by her. I soon disabused her of that notion and amended the relevant parts she marked on my "co-operation card".' It is not just that hospital care is sometimes stark and unfriendly; many women feel that the failure to achieve any continuity actually results in second-class or dangerous medicine and obstetrics.

The pregnant woman has a responsibility, for herself and her baby, to discover the choices open to her, weigh their relative advantages, and make sure that everybody knows what she wants. It means that she also has to be sufficiently courageous to complain when necessary and to withdraw her consent for procedures that she is not happy about unless more convincing arguments are produced. This is very different from the traditional feminine role, and many women feel acutely uncomfortable with it. They want to please; it feels good to make the doctor smile; they do not want to fuss or, indeed, to be noticed as different in any way. It is much easier to conform to the doctor's expectations of the 'good patient'. Diana Scully, in her study of the training of obstetricians and gynaecologists in the United States,[4] asked doctors how they would describe a good patient. Their answers emphasized passivity, obedience and middle-class status. One said: 'The main thing is that the patient understands what I say, listens to what I say, does what I say, believes what I say.'

The 'vocal minority'

A woman who has had the opportunity of education and a career has special responsibilities in this because she is speaking for other women who have not had her advantages and who may be even more confused and anxious than she is. Yet she has to be prepared for possible hostility or suspicion on the part of the doctor simply because she is an 'educated' woman asking questions. (In the past, the medical press has sometimes labelled such women the 'vocal minority'.) A doctor has often been trained to see pregnant women only as patients who receive instructions, and may think of skills of communication as giving these instructions clearly, rather than as a two-way conversation. If the patient does not comply, she is 'a defaulter'.

Ann Oakley, in her book *Subject Women*,[5] writes:

> The idea that it is women who cause the deaths of babies – by not going to antenatal clinics (or not going early enough), by smoking, eating the wrong food, having sexual intercourse, not being married . . . implicitly acknowledges women's disobedience in doing what they think is best for themselves and their babies.

So it is often difficult to talk with doctors and get them to listen to you. Few doctors today would openly state, as did one in the 1970s to a patient who questioned his diagnosis, 'I will tell you what is wrong with you, I will tell you what your symptoms are, and I will tell you what to do. I am the doctor and you will kindly not forget the fact.'[6] But there are probably many doctors who come very near to such an outburst, especially when a pregnant woman is insistent about the kind of care she would like, and how she wants the birth to be.

It helps to have access to really good published epidemiological research which presents the results of randomized, controlled trials of obstetric interventions. One source for this information is the two-volume *Effective Care in Pregnancy and Childbirth*[7]. Any woman who questions treatment on the basis of something she has read may be dismissed with 'You mustn't believe everything you read' or castigated with the shocked discovery, 'You've been reading books!'

There are, of course, universities where psychology and the acquisition of interview techniques form part of medical courses. But even these skills may be used as a means of acquiring power over patients and manipulating them effectively. A professor of obstetrics, describing the advances in the teaching of medical students in his own department, told me, 'We have a film on how to deal with a difficult patient.' (We are still awaiting, unfortunately, the film on how to deal with a difficult doctor.) He went on to explain some of the techniques of interviewing that were taught: 'Eye contact is important,' he said and, fixing me with an unwavering glare, added, 'You will notice that I am making eye contact with you now.'

Doctors now also learn to see pregnant women as 'consumers', and to take patient satisfaction into the reckoning. According to this paradigm, pregnant women are like shoppers allowed to choose between brands of washing detergent or to select cakes in a well-presented display. But suppose they do not want cakes in the first place? It is the duty of the store manager to see that they do.

Women are not just consumers of health care. In childbirth we are the producers, without whom the doctors would have no jobs. Women should be able to say what they want, and – unless it can be shown through properly conducted research that this would be positively dangerous – expect it to be provided.

It is not only a question of expressing feelings. It is often claimed that all pregnant women are emotionally vulnerable. Perhaps. But this is no excuse for treating them as incapable of rational thought, or so concerned with their own emotions that they are 'selfish and egotistical', and cannot be trusted to consider their babies' needs.[8] The opposite is nearer the truth. Women who want loving people around them in labour, who criticize excessive intervention in childbirth, or decline drugs, those who seek home birth or water birth, or insist that they are not separated from their newborn babies, do these things *because* they want what is best for their babies, are concerned about their babies' safety and well-being, and are thinking about how they would like to welcome them into the world.

Being 'high risk'

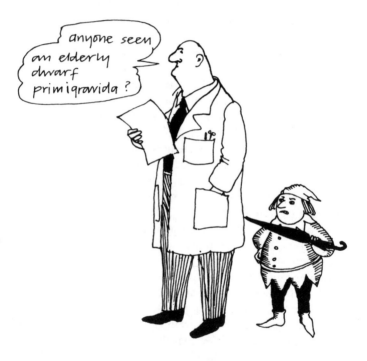

anyone seen an elderly dwarf primigravida?

As we have seen, the older woman may find that she is in a 'high-risk' category simply because of her age. For some obstetricians, this classification includes all first-time mothers over 30. Others tend to include in this category only women of 35 and older. A few believe that it should include women having first babies at 28. Different terms are used to describe them. 'Elderly primigravida' is one, which, as one woman said, 'made me feel very long in the tooth'. A woman who was 5 feet tall was very alarmed at being categorized as an 'elderly *dwarf* primigravida'. A 'gravida' is simply a pregnant woman. So a 'multigravida' is one who has had previous pregnancies. If you are pregnant but have had two previous miscarriages, you are a 'gravida'. The other term is 'parity' to describe the number of previous pregnancies that have gone through to 28 weeks or beyond. If you are 'para 3' you have had three births. If you are 'para 3 + 1' you have had three births and one miscarriage. Multiple births and miscarriages are counted as one in this system of reckoning. A 'nulliparous' woman is one who is having her first pregnancy, though the terms 'primigravida' or 'primipara' are often used loosely instead.

There is no reason to think that birth will be more painful or difficult because you are over 35. Many women in their late thirties and forties are healthier than they have ever been because they care for themselves, understand their bodies, and ensure that they get exercise and have a good diet. A healthy woman of 40 is in much better condition for labour than an unhealthy one in her twenties.

It may also be that a woman has more stamina and courage than when she was younger. An experienced midwife, Ina May Gaskin, says that women over 35 are unlikely to 'waste time and precious energy during labour by feeling sorry for themselves or by fighting labour'. She claims that, 'a woman with a mature attitude is usually able to use the energy of labour efficiently, to rest effectively while dilating, or in between pushes'. She thinks it is ridiculous to consider entire categories of women as high-risk simply because of their age, and accuses doctors of 'a very crude and unscientific brand of obstetrics'.[9]

The perinatal mortality rate (PMR)

Statistically, risks to the baby are higher for women giving birth over 30 than for those in their twenties. Under 20, the risks are also higher. The perinatal mortality rate (PMR) is a record of deaths of babies at birth or in the week following. The figure is given as a proportion per 1,000 births. In England and Wales, for example, the PMR in 1991 was about 8 per 1,000. This is a crude figure, however, because it does not tell us anything about the quality of life of the babies who live or about the mothers who are most likely to have babies who die. One of the most significant facts about the British PMR is that it is almost twice as safe to have a baby if you are married to a man in a profession or in management than if you are at the bottom of the social scale, married to someone in an unskilled occupation or who is unemployed. (All these figures are based on the occupation of the partner.) Women who are unsupported are at greatest risk of all. It is clear that perinatal mortality reflects poverty. It stems from all the things we associate with social disadvantage: lack of education, poor housing, overcrowding, inadequate nutrition, stress, environmental poisons, and perhaps also simply from not being able to operate the 'system', being powerless and unable even to claim social security benefits.

It is difficult to isolate these variables because being poor brings with it many other disadvantages for the foetus. Smoking in pregnancy is more common. Some eight deaths in every 1,000 births might be avoided if women did not smoke when pregnant, and many more babies would survive with better birth weights. Congenital malformations such as spina bifida, including those that are incompatible with life, are also more frequent at the bottom of the social scale, and these alone account for 22 per cent of perinatal deaths. Some 70 per cent of babies who die do so because they are born prematurely. Here again there is an association with social class. The higher the social class, the lower the percentage of preterm births. The poor may live in heavily built-up inner-city areas where lead from car exhausts pollutes the air. If a woman is at the bottom of the social scale she is more likely to get pregnant while still in her teens, and some women who cannot cope with contraception, or whose partners are unwilling to, go on having babies when they are themselves in poor health. There is also a continuum of disadvantage; though individuals break out of the pattern, it tends to be passed on from parents to children. There is mounting evidence that it is important that a woman has good nutrition, not during pregnancy, but before. This reflects the social-class culture in which she lives and perhaps also that in which she was reared. Her nutrition while she was growing up may be another factor in the equation, and perhaps even her own parents' nutrition.

The upshot of all this is that if you are reading this page, then the statistics of highest risk, stemming from poor social conditions, are very unlikely to apply to you. If you are willing to terminate a pregnancy should foetal disability be diagnosed, risk is still further reduced. In good health yourself with a straightforward pregnancy in which no special risk factors are detected, you can expect a normal labour and a healthy baby. There is no such thing as 'no risk'. After all, even crossing a road looking both ways has its risks. Generalizations that older mothers always have difficult births, that an older woman's baby after a normal pregnancy is at greater risk, or that older mothers are less successful at breastfeeding, are untrue.

It is difficult to measure pain or guess whether the birth is likely to be more (or less) painful because of your age, because so much depends on your attitude of mind, and whether you feel that pain is *attacking* you or working *for* you. This in itself is influenced by the environment in which birth takes place, by psychological factors such as whether or not you feel cherished and emotionally supported, and by such things as tiredness or exhaustion and conflicting emotions about what is happening. All these affect the perception of pain. One woman who delivered in the bath at home, comfortably lapped in warm water, commented:

> I do not want to give the impression that it was all dream-like pleasure. Obviously if it had not been for the birth of our baby, the same sensations would have been painful. Only the love and joy transformed the contractions into a 'labour' rather than a 'pain'.

Induced labour

Some obstetricians have a policy of inducing labour – starting it artificially – in all their patients over a certain age. A doctor will sometimes tell the woman in early pregnancy, 'I won't let you go past your date at your age', or tell her to come into hospital a week, or even two weeks, *before* she is due, to be induced. Even if you have a *medical* condition, the most common of which is diabetes, an obstetrician cannot possibly tell while you are still in the first half of pregnancy whether you can be induced safely with no risk to your baby. In spite of modern methods of estimating gestation such as serial ultrasound, mistakes can be made about the age of the foetus, and babies are still induced and delivered before they are ready for life, with consequent breathing problems.

The length of pregnancy is assumed to be 280 days or 40 weeks, often regardless of the length of the menstrual cycle. This results from a linear model of thinking. It is as if time is stretched in a long line and we have to count it out in separate sections. This shapes ideas of when labour should start, how long it should last, and the time that dilatation and expulsion should take. Anything else is considered abnormal.[10] When periods have been irregular it is especially difficult to know when ovulation occurred. Some 30 per cent of babies are delivered before the estimated date and 70 per cent after the date. Most pregnancies last anything between 38 and 42 weeks, though 90 per cent of births take place within ten days of the due date. Your age is an insufficient reason for inducing labour. In the United States, the average length of pregnancy is no longer than 40 weeks. It is 38 weeks because of the high rate of induction.

Induction should only be performed after you have discussed the reasons for it, having been given accurate information, had time to think about it, been told exactly what happens, and given your consent in writing. Otherwise you may want to give your informed *refusal*. It is easier for you to consider the matter if you are out of hospital, in your normal surroundings. Some doctors expect patients to agree on the spot, or send them into an adjoining room for a few minutes to make up their minds. You can say, 'I'd like more time to think about this, and I don't think I can let you know before next Tuesday', or 'I want time to talk this over with my partner', though the doctor may then ask, 'Is your partner an obstetrician?' and, if you say 'no', may say, 'Well, how can he possibly help you decide, then?' – which is what happened to one woman of 36.

Your antenatal teacher may be a good person with whom to discuss possible induction. She knows what happens and will probably know which obstetricians perform it most readily, and if they tend to pressurize their patients into it or suggest that the baby will die if the induction does not go ahead. Some obstetricians regularly make their patients in late pregnancy feel emotionally blackmailed. Women say that they are asked, 'Are you prepared to accept responsibility if your baby dies?' or 'You do realize you are risking your baby's life, don't you?'

Though your childbirth teacher can give you information, she is usually torn between providing the facts so that you can decide yourself, and making things as easy and comfortable as possible for you so that whatever happens you are able to adapt to labour. She may feel, 'If this woman is going to have an induced labour anyway I can help her accept it psychologically and reassure her about what happens.' And she is quite right if she tells you that some women have very happy, straightforward induced labours. On the other hand, many do not. Though techniques of induction have improved in most hospitals since then, I did a study of women's experiences of induction[11] that revealed that women being induced need far more painkillers. Some 95 per cent of women who had attended National Childbirth Trust antenatal classes had drugs for pain relief when labour was induced. Women who go to classes often hope to manage without drugs as far as possible. When labour was not induced, 50 per cent coped without them. Those women who had already had babies with a non-induced labour were asked to compare the induced labour with the previous labour that was not induced. Usually second births are easier than the first. The majority of these women said that the second birth was *more* painful.

The babies did not do so well either, though more babies of induced labours were probably at risk for other reasons. A much larger proportion of newborns were separated from their mothers because they were put in the intensive care nursery. These babies were unlikely all to have been ill, since policy used to be to put every baby delivered after a difficult labour under the watchful eyes of the intensive care sister just in case. Since the publication of the work of Klaus and Kennell on bonding,[12] this policy has been changed in many hospitals.

Because of analgesics the mothers had taken there was also another kind of separation. Many women experienced a *pharmacological* separation from their babies, whom they could not hold because they felt too 'woozy' or could not see because they fell asleep. This separation severely affected the first meeting between mother and baby immediately following birth and for several hours afterwards. It also affected breastfeeding, since the time when the baby can most naturally and easily go to the mother's breast after birth was missed. Many of the babies were knocked out by the drugs the mother had taken. This was usually pethidine, or pethidine in combination with other drugs.

Once labour is induced and the bag of waters has been ruptured, there is no way back. The obstetrician is committed to getting you delivered within 24 hours. To wait any longer than this increases the risk of infection. He has to be prepared, therefore, to engage in 'active management' to keep to a timetable. Professor Ian Donald warned that 'any intervention, however apparently trivial, carries with it the responsibilities for consequence . . .'[13] The decision to induce labour is as serious a one as a decision to perform a Caesarean section. The rate of intravenous oxytocin can be stepped up to make the uterus work harder. This causes more pain, so pethidine or an epidural may be offered before or shortly after. If the cervix fails to dilate quickly or the baby reacts with type two dips in its heart rate – ones that persist after the contraction has ended – the obstetrician will be ready to intervene with Caesarean section. If the cervix dilates but there is a hold-up then, because the woman has an epidural and cannot feel how to push, or is too doped or exhausted to do so, delivery can be accomplished by forceps or vacuum extraction, or with a Caesarean. Induced labours are more likely to finish with forceps[14, 15] or Caesarean[16] deliveries.

Failed induction

An induction that ends in a Caesarean section is a *failed* induction. Some 2 per cent upwards of all inductions end in a Caesarean. Professor Donald warned: 'No method of induction is both absolutely certain and safe.'[17] In the United Kingdom induction was most in vogue in the early 1970s. At that time, nearly 40 per cent of all labours were induced. The rate has fallen since then, largely because it has been discovered that high induction rates do not save babies' lives. But there is still wide variation between different hospitals and even inside the same hospital between different consultants. You can ask the obstetrician the induction rate in the hospital. If it is below 15 per cent, listen to the explanation of why you need to be induced with great care because there will be good reasons. If it is over 25 per cent, labours are probably being induced unnecessarily. Between these two figures there is a grey area, because hospitals in different cities care for women coming from widely varying backgrounds and high-risk women from poor social backgrounds *may* benefit from more intervention than women who have no known risk factors. In fact, studies reveal that poor women get *less* intervention than women who are better off.[18]

It is widely believed that since the induction 'scare' of the 1970s induction rates have plummeted. This is not so. Even where fewer inductions are done, acceleration of labours that have already started is common. This practice, too, has its risks, which are much the same as those of induction. Some obstetricians believe that it is right to actively manage the labours of all first-time mothers over 35. It is more difficult to resist an intravenous drip of synthetic oxytocin once you are already in hospital and in bed. But no intervention should take place unless you have it explained and have agreed to it. In practice, once a patient has been told about a procedure in however rudimentary a way (in response to 'I'm going to give you a bit of help now', or 'I'm just going to give you a little prick', one woman – usually refined – exclaimed, 'I don't care whether your prick is big or little. I don't want it!') it is taken for granted that she has understood and accepted the intervention. So you have to be quick to say, 'No thank you' or 'Hold on! I'd like to discuss this'.

Induction should be done in two circumstances: when the baby is obviously safer out than in because the intra-uterine environment is poor; and when the mother's health is going to suffer severely if the pregnancy continues. The cervix should be ripe. If it is not, in some countries prostaglandin pessaries can be used overnight or some hours in advance to ripen it before the infusion of oxytocin is started. Sometimes oxytocin is unnecessary as labour proceeds with prosta-glandin alone. This is much more comfortable for the mother, and may allow labour to progress more normally because she can be up and about.

If you are induced, do not expect labour to be rapid. It can be long drawn out, and the so-called latent phase, before there is effective dila-tation of the cervix, may be prolonged.

Similarly, if a Caesarean section is recommended, though the news comes as a shock, take time to discuss the pros and cons with your doctor. It may be that a trial of labour, with everything ready for a Caesarean section if necessary, is a better idea. In many cases no one knows for sure what a uterus can do until contractions have got under way. Giving yourself a chance of avoiding a Caesarean is safe even if you have had three or more sections previously. Eighty-nine women who had had at least one Caesarean tried for VBAC (vaginal birth after Caesarean section), and 771 had an elective Caesarean. There were no cases of maternal morbidity (uterine rupture, bladder or bowel injury, laceration of the uterine artery, blood transfusion and fever) and those who had had three or more previous Caesareans had similar success – a vaginal birth – to those who had already had one and those delivered by elective repeat section.[19] If it proves to be a Caesarean after all, consider one with epidural anaesthesia. This enables you to be awake when your baby is born and aware of everything that is going on. Abby said it was

> fantastic! They erected a green curtain across my tum so I couldn't see. I felt no pain, only pressure. Then as soon as they delivered the baby they lowered the curtain and gave her to me. I fell in love with her straight away. We were lost in wonder over our new daughter.

Fathers are often present at a Caesarean under epidural, and this is worth asking for. If an obstetrician has not had a father there before he may find it helpful and reassuring to meet your partner beforehand, and may be willing to try it as an experiment with someone he already knows.

Self-doubt

Seeds of self-doubt are sometimes sown inadvertently in an older woman's mind during pregnancy by other people's remarks. You laugh them off at the time, but in the middle of the night they sprout. One woman of 38 said that the pregnant teenagers in the hospital were 'aghast' when they learned her age and exclaimed, 'You're old enough to be my mum!' and 'My God! You never imagine teachers having babies!' Older mothers often mention remarks made by doctors like, 'You're a bit old for this sort of thing, aren't you?' or 'We'll have to keep an eye on you'. One woman was lying on the examination table with her lower half exposed when the senior obstetrician swept in, followed by a retinue of students, notebooks poised. 'Ah!' exclaimed the great man, 'here we have the perfect example of an elderly primigravida!'

'And a talking elderly primigravida too!' said the patient, raising her head.

If an expectant mother tries to talk about avoiding episiotomy – a cut made to enlarge the birth outlet – she may feel accused of deliberately intending to injure her baby by making the birth difficult for it, and threatened with postnatal sexual problems and the consequent breakdown of a sexual relationship, and by prolapse later in life unless she agrees to one. The obstetricians genuinely believe that their way is better than nature's and can offer improved and what Sir John Dewhurst – a former President of the Royal College of Gynaecologists and Obstetricians – calls 'enhanced' childbirth. Such obstetricians are sincere and often deeply committed to their beliefs. When you discuss your treatment with them, bear this in mind.

In spite of feeling vulnerable and at a disadvantage with her underwear off, an older woman really does have more chance of getting the doors of communication open with the doctors, even if they often need a bit of a shove. She may be of the same age as those caring for her, so they have that in common, or the doctor may be younger so that she does not feel in awe of him.

A sense of humour helps, if only because the woman who insists on knowing what is being done to her and why is readily labelled as 'anxious', 'neurotic' or 'difficult' and this may be written into her notes. If you can be firm and persistent, but at the same time keep a light touch, you give yourself more chance of genuine 'rapport'. If you have a male partner, taking him with you to meet the obstetrician means that he not only appreciates what you go through at the clinic, but can ask questions too. It may also put the obstetrician more at ease, as some hospital doctors do not like talking to women and find it much simpler to talk 'man to man'. If you do this you have to be sure that the two will not start colluding together, however, and make decisions *for* you. Get as much information as you can, talk through together in advance the things that matter most to you, and make notes of priorities. You might even try acting out a hypothetical discussion, taking it in turns to play the part of the obstetrician. If the answer to a question is unconvincing, how are you going to follow it up? Remember that you do not have to come to any snap decisions. Unless there is a dire emergency you can always take time to think things through. Just say, 'I'd like time to think about that'.

Talk with your doctor as a human being, not as an authoritarian professional in a white coat. (Think of him in his pyjamas!) And bear in mind that many obstetricians are rushed, overworked and under great pressure because they see far too many patients in too short a time. This

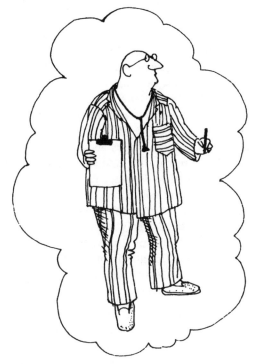

Think of your doctor in his pyjamas

does not mean that you should not take your time to talk because you are thinking of the other patients waiting (though that is a natural reaction), but that you need to think ahead as to what you want to say, use the interview constructively, and *thank* him or her for giving you the time. Sheer pressure of numbers sometimes means that you have to put off a discussion until another time. In some clinics doctors spend on average just two minutes with each patient. Explain that this discussion is important to you and make at least an unofficial appointment for it. If you cannot get anyone to make time for you, write a letter to the obstetrician. Once something is in the records it tends to be noticed, if only because it is open to other people's perusal too.

A woman may choose a female doctor – one who has had babies herself – because she thinks it will be easier to talk to her. Some women obstetricians understand just how disempowering the medical system can be because they have experienced this themselves, and have not become sucked into the medical establishment. But you cannot assume that because your obstetrician – or, for that matter, your GP – is a woman, she shares any of your views about birth. Women in obstetrics have to struggle for recognition and status against a system that is heavily dominated by men. To do this, they often copy men. It may be the only route to success in their careers.

Some of the problems older mothers encounter in pregnancy and labour result from the obstetrician's concern about them and too much doctoring, rather than from any inherent condition. Pregnancy is seen primarily not as a natural physiological state, but as a hazardous process. Judith Lumley, a lecturer in obstetrics in Australia, puts it this way:

> The distinction between normal and abnormal pregnancy has become blurred. Some doctors reject the 'normal' as inappropriate, and classify all pregnant women as low-risk, medium-risk or high-risk patients. Normality becomes an accolade, to be bestowed after the event on the few women who pass through pregnancy and birth without deviating from the physiological ideal at any point.[20]

In this the older pregnant woman, especially one having a baby for the first time, has all the odds stacked against her. Obstetric and midwifery textbooks sometimes discuss her as if she had one foot in the grave, with increased chances of uterine fibroids, miscarriage, hypertension, premature labour, long, dysfunctional labour, forceps delivery and Caesarean section. It is understandable that the doctor who does not have much experience of the normal, healthy older pregnant woman may become anxious and then convey the anxiety to the patient. When a woman's blood pressure goes up, for example, this may be a direct result of a proliferation of investigations that threaten confidence, warnings from doctors, and fraught attendances at the childbirth clinic. She goes in feeling happy and fit and comes out feeling reproductively incompetent and sick with fear, frustration and, often, suppressed anger. It would be surprising if this did *not* have an effect on her blood pressure.

Keeping calm

It may help to build some calm into your daily life: yoga, meditation, relaxation or a space for slow full breathing, or simply luxuriating in a leisurely bath in a darkened room. Finding a way to express what you feel is also vital. Anger is legitimate, and it can help to cry, shout or bash the pillows. Most women try to go on as if nothing had happened and to be 'reasonable', thus giving implicit acceptance to the assumption that anything can be required of a woman *for the sake of the baby*. Objecting to the way you are being treated seems selfish, since it is all being done for your baby.

A 38-year-old woman who is herself a midwife came to realize halfway through her pregnancy that she wanted a home birth:

> I felt, 'I can't leave this house. I need to give birth in my own space.' I told my doctor, who was horrified. She upset me a lot. She told me that the baby would die. She was totally unco-operative, but two of my best friends are the best midwives around – so I simply bypassed her.

When things go badly wrong, if a doctor lacks any understanding of your experience, there are failures in communication, or care becomes abusive, write to complain both to the doctor concerned and to the relevant authority. A woman who had the Triple Test was informed that she had a one in seventy chance of a Down's syndrome baby. Her doctor, rather than discussing with her arrangements for amniocentesis, took it for granted that she would have an abortion, and booked a hospital bed for it. When the woman said that she did not plan on having an abortion the doctor replied, 'Oh well, Down's syndrome children can be very affectionate – like dogs.' She made an official complaint.

Some older women have relatively good experiences of care, especially those who have careers in the health service. They feel on familiar ground and may know those caring for them. Others enjoy being part of the workings of an efficiently run institution and are secure and confident with the application of modern technology to the business of childbirth. Fiona says that her 'present idea of heaven would be to spend a week in hospital, enjoying anonymity, gloriously free from domestic demands and the company of my (albeit loving) family'. With a side-slash at my own views, she adds: 'Some women are not so Luddite as to be thrown into hysteria at the site of gleaming machinery.' Even she, however, describes one incident in her happy hospital experience in which she felt completely depersonalized. She was being pushed out of the delivery room on a trolley and up to the ward in a lift, surrounded by porters and nurses: 'They were joking about their weekend dates and I wondered if it would be rude to join in the conversation. But it became clear to me that it wasn't expected. I was simply a body in transit.'

It takes an effort of will and imagination to move on from that situation to accept that care-givers can be collaborators rather than powerful authority figures appropriating from us the responsibility for the outcome of the pregnancy. Though a distorted medical perspective often implies that statistics ought to rule our lives, personal experience tells us that such a view of life is untenable. The value we attach to particular events and qualities of relationships must also affect the decisions we make. If we thought only in terms of statistics and reducing the perinatal mortality by one more decimal point, no matter what effect this had on human emotions and values, we could make it a matter of public policy to detect all multiple pregnancies by ultrasound and abort them immediately since these babies are likely to be born preterm and be low birth weight. That we do not abort all twins and triplets shows that values do not depend on mere arithmetic. Even doctors most passionately concerned about perinatal mortality statistics have not proposed this solution. Nor can we ever have *complete* safety in childbirth. Expecting a baby to be perfect if you do all the right things and have every available investigation sets an impossibly high, unrealistic standard. As more and more tests for foetal well-being are devised, the situation may develop in which the older expectant mother could spend much of her time undergoing procedures of one kind or another. The decision as to how much to probe and investigate is not a medical matter in the long run, but has to do with the quality of life and how much intervention we are prepared to tolerate for the sake of more knowledge. The pursuit of perfection in human reproduction is a mirage.

Ross Mitchell of the Department of Child Health at Dundee University expressed it this way:

In human reproduction, the analogy of the production line or conveyor belt is inappropriate: it implies a uniform, repeatable, and flawless standard of product, anything less than this being instantly and rightly rejected. In laying too great emphasis on the goal of faultless excellence, we may have done a misservice to some children and their parents. Every person is the result of many interacting influences, some beneficial and others inimical to development. The mother's anxious scrutiny of her new baby to assure herself that he is unblemished and her overreaction to the slightest deviation from an ideal norm are intensified by the tacit professional assumption that perfection is the yardstick.[21]

6

Life after the baby comes

When you are still pregnant it is very difficult to summon the imaginative energy to think about how things may be after the baby arrives. Discussions about how you might feel, for instance, seem purely academic. The birth is the all-important challenge. Yet for many women that fourth trimester of pregnancy, the three months after birth, its delights and difficulties, are more exciting, exhausting and deeply satisfying than even the birth itself. You are bucketed out of a peak emotional experience straight into an activity and commitment that keeps you at full stretch almost 24 hours a day. First-time mothers say:

> The most devastating thing is that once the child is born it is a total stranger. You have some idea of the times it will wake and sleep from the times it has been kicking you to bits, but otherwise you know nothing about it. This is frightening.

> I felt I was a feeding and changing machine. The constant physical and emotional involvement with a dependent small human being was such a contrast to my previous life as a librarian in an academic library. I realized how unprepared I was. Watching a health visitor bathe a doll is a far cry from the real thing.

> I had awful depression on the third day. Difficult because Robert (my husband) was still physically and emotionally exhausted. He's not used to feeling so much so intensely. We yelled at each other and I cried and wanted to die – about what we're going to eat for dinner, for goodness sake! The midwife was worried and asked her relief to come the next day – to find me up and about singing and washing nappies.

> Having been a teacher used to dealing with about thirty-five children I thought I'd find a baby a piece of cake. Although I was on a 'high', I still found those first six weeks totally exhausting. I fell in love with my daughter from the first second I saw her. It really was like being in love. Every time I woke up I'd be overwhelmed with excitement – yes, even at three in the morning. I loved being

with her, near her, touching her, kissing her, looking at her and thinking constantly of her.

The responsibility for this new life can be frightening. A woman who has been anxiously trying to fit the whole business of having a baby and rearing it into her own well-organized lifestyle may sometimes feel as if the ground has opened beneath her. The conflict between her career goals, her desires, and the demands of her own ego and the over-whelming pull of the baby's needs produces grotesque and disturbing fantasies, both night-time dreams and day-time images that have the quality of hallucinations. A woman who had taken steps to be sterilized before she decided she wanted to have a baby was deeply troubled by the sense of her power to avoid pregnancy. It was as if she were the bad queen or wicked witch of the story books:

> Every night since I came home from hospital I have woken up not knowing where she is, thinking that she's in the bed, or believing that she's been squashed or suffocated. Sometimes the disturbance is quite mild and John tells me that she's in her room. At the other extreme, I have woken up crying out and desperately searching for her under the pillows.

There is also the astonishing reality of the baby, not just a package but a person. Many women feel the wave of passionate love that enthrals them is so intense that it makes it difficult to cope in the 'real' world, with its lunch and supper times, daily routines, dealing with visitors, the questions and the demands of relationships and people's expecta-tions of you.

Sylvia Plath expressed vividly this joy even though depression finally conquered her, and suggests the strength of the complete giving of oneself to the baby in her poem:

> What did my fingers do before they held him?
> What did my heart do with its love?
> I have never seen a thing so dear.
> His lids are like the lilac-flower
> And soft as a moth, his breath.
> I shall not let go.[1]

If you have already had a baby, even ten years ago, you know all about this and can smile in recollection; you think back to the feelings of utter incompetence, perhaps, the awful self-doubts, the panic, the emotional swings, the sweetness as the baby lay sleeping peacefully, the awesome responsibility of protecting and caring for this new life, the firmness of the rounded limbs against your body, the heaviness of the head as a feed finished in utter content, the fine down on the skin and the scent of warm peaches.

A whetted appetite

Women having another baby after a long space, though they may feel aghast at what they have done, and at the beginning of pregnancy be resentful about being, as one woman said, 'put back firmly in the home' and 'trapped', look forward to these things with a whetted appetite. They know it will be crazy and chaotic, but it is going to be fun! It is not just a question of the baby 'keeping you young' either; it may feel, once the baby is really there, as if the choice is between rejuvenation and collapse.

The mother of a 'surprise' baby often feels a special passionate closeness to the child. One said that this was 'almost psychic'. 'Perhaps,' she added, 'we have to fight for their entry into this world that much more and the fight has provided the bond.' She had considered abortion and, after a struggle, had decided firmly against it, in the face of other people's advice. One battle for this particular woman was against the horrified disapproval of her own mother, who would not speak to her for six months. Many women also feel the hurdles of tests through which they go during pregnancy are also like part of a long struggle to have the baby.

When the older woman compares her experience with the late-born baby with how she was as a mother with earlier children, she always says how much more relaxed, confident and at ease she is this time round. Motherhood is not just a matter of biology. Her attitude of mind is vital – the spirit in which she starts out on this new adventure. Women with a second family have a different time scale from even those older mothers who are having first-born children, and say they spend time with the baby because everything else seems relatively unimportant: 'I know that time passes all too quickly when children are small,' one mother, previously in educational research, remarks, 'and that these early years are crucial for future learning, social behaviour and exploration.' The experienced mother also realizes that problems that seem insurmountable at the time all pass before long. One who felt 'cloistered' with her baby during feeds that went on and on and on, remembered this stage was a temporary one, and reflected that she needed this time to get to know her baby properly and to protect herself from outside stresses.

For the first-time mother over 35, the initial challenges appear rather different. Looking ahead to the enforced change of role, the excitement is mixed with anxiety, not just about coping, but about what the baby's arrival will do to her as a person. For a time it is delightful not to have to rush out and be 'bright and interesting', but even while she basks in this satisfaction there may be stirrings of restlessness. This is intensified if the baby is at first unwanted. As one woman, commenting on the distress she experienced after the birth of her baby, said:

> I lost my personal space. My overriding preoccupation is how I am going to get back to work. At first I thought I'd probably have to give up work and felt very resentful of the baby. It was a tremendous upheaval to discover I was pregnant. I have a fantastic doctor and he made a lot of time to talk so that I didn't bottle this up inside. I decided, yes, I do want to have the baby. Now I'm anxious about how we are going to get along. Will we like each other? How are we going to sort this one out together?

Her opportunity to talk freely with her doctor helped her move from concern solely with what the birth of the baby was going to do to *her* to fascination about her relationship with this new person. Without the opportunity to talk, that progression might have been delayed until well after the baby came.

A career crisis

For a career woman, having a baby provokes a crisis that she often realizes may never be resolved. One new mother, completely committed to her career and unwilling to take time out from it, said her mind was only set at rest when her obstetrician stated, 'Right! I promise to keep you working as long as I can and get you back to work as soon as possible after.' Many women are far less sure that this is what they want. They do not know whether they will want to go back to work or, if they intend to do so, how soon they and the baby will be ready for this. Shall it be job only, baby only, or job and baby? Within the EU, it is now law that a woman cannot be dismissed from her job because of pregnancy. In October 2010 the European Parliament decided that all companies should pay maternity leave at full pay for 20 weeks and paternity leave for two weeks. Previously women would receive 90 per cent of their salary for the first six weeks of leave, followed by the statutory rate of £125.00 per week for the remaining 46 weeks. A woman must be able to return to her previous job within 29 weeks of the birth if she indicated before she took maternity leave that she wanted her job back.

The decision as to whether, in fact, you want it back lies with you – and you can change your mind at any time. If you say you do not want to return, however, you are closing the door on the options open to you.

A pregnant woman may be very uncertain of what her feelings are going to be after the baby arrives, and perhaps does not trust that she is ever going to fall in love with her baby. 'Your career is about to take off or is already well established,' Tricia explained. 'For me it was the problem of when to break, and that if I did have two or three years out it would be difficult to get back in.' Virginia said she planned to do a post-graduate degree to 'keep her mind awake', and was afraid that having a baby would fuddle her brain unless she took determined steps to develop new career skills.

Financial problems may loom large, not because of an overall shortage of money, but because a woman in her thirties is usually earning more than she did ten years before, and the disappearance of one partner's salary makes a dramatic difference. She is often anxious about the loss of independence and freedom that comes from having her own income:

> Thinking of being financially dependent on my partner upsets me. I've been independent for so long. I feel trapped by the thought that I have to ask for money for the everyday things of life, having to say, 'Please can I have some money because I can't get through this month?' or 'Would you mind paying the electricity bill?'

A woman who says she is 'lucky' because she works two hours a day at home designing children's clothes says that without this and her own money she would feel frustrated. The independence that is being fought for is more than economic. For many women it expresses anxiety about loss of selfhood.

The fear is that you are going to be somehow sucked in by baby care, your brain will turn to a vegetable, and you will become just 'a mother'. A woman to whom children are stuck like 'barnacles encrusting a ship and limpets clinging to a rock' is the awful image summoned up by Margaret Atwood in *The Edible Woman*.[2] For the committed feminist there is the inherent threat that she has 'sold out' to motherhood and to a role stereotype that legitimizes the social inferiority of women. One woman said that her feminist friends 'are upset at my loss of independence, and opting out'.

First-time mothers look very carefully at their friends and relations who have small children. They watch them with all the vigilance and concentration of an ethnologist observing a pack of orang-utans. And they tend to come away highly critical of what they see.

Total devotion?

A group of pregnant women having first babies in their thirties were discussing the kind of mothers they hoped to be. They were all anxious about devoting themselves entirely to the baby:

'I know a couple who haven't been out to dinner with each other for eighteen months,' Maureen said.

'It's the same with some friends of ours,' said another. 'But it's a very awkward baby. It won't sleep for longer than three hours and she is just so tired.'

Julia said: 'I get rather cross at the relish with which other women say, "Oh, you won't have a minute to yourself, and you won't have time to read a book." They seem to enjoy saying this. I just cannot imagine not having time to read or write a letter. I can't imagine being so tired. It makes me very depressed.'

'From some of the things people say,' Jan exclaimed, 'I get the feeling that I'm expected to metamorphose into a completely different person. Two friends who are doctors and who were at the peaks of their careers said, "It's wonderful to vegetate at home". I don't think it will be. I have a fear that something biological will happen to me.'

Another woman remarked that even during her pregnancy friends seem to be distancing themselves: 'It's almost as if being pregnant is supposed to affect your decision-making and therefore your opinions are not worth listening to.'

The contrast between these anxieties and the surge of emotion that comes with being a new mother is startling. The woman no longer seems to be protecting herself in the same way. Joan, a nurse for 20 years, who had her first baby at 38, said she feared that she had thrown away her last vestige of independence for ever when she became pregnant. She went on to describe her emotional journey into motherhood. After a difficult and painful 17-hour labour she had a forceps delivery and her baby was taken immediately to the special care baby unit:

I confess I was relieved not to have to look after him the first night as I was deeply shocked by all the pain. But during the days that followed I was filled with pure delight at this little person who I found hard to believe was really mine. I appreciate that having babies is old hat to most people and there is nothing unique about my experience, but the feelings that came to me so unexpectedly were ones of overwhelming emotion for which I felt I had been ill-prepared. Sometimes I was torn apart by the thought that something might happen to the baby. He meant much more to me than I had imagined.

Bonding

In the mid-1970s two paediatricians became fascinated by the emotional intensity of which they became aware as they observed mothers with their newborn babies, and analysed what went on between them.[3] Doctors had discovered mother love. They started to learn about the dialogue that begins within seconds of birth when a woman is able to hold her newborn baby and gaze into his or her eyes. Systems that attempt to facilitate this process have now been incorporated into care in many hospitals in the West. It is called 'bonding'. Care-givers are supposed to allow time for it, check that it is occurring, and in some hospitals to record this on the patient's chart.

The medical takeover of mother love involves the use of ultrasound in pregnancy, too. Observing that mothers are surprised, delighted and intrigued when they 'see' their babies on the ultrasound screen, some obstetricians assert that this should be included as a routine part of care to enable women to fall in love with their babies. Love is too important to be left to mothers it seems! It must be 'integrated' into obstetric management.[4] Yet mothers have eagerly reached out their arms for their babies, and have fallen passionately in love with them, for thousands of years before doctors sought to take control of this emotional transformation. Indeed, if it becomes – like dilatation of the cervix and the length of the first and second stages of labour – a process that is medically managed, there is a real risk that doctors may do more harm than good.

The emotions that flood in as the baby is lifted out of your body are often unexpected and seem to have no connection with more conventional ideas of love. Some older women who have had no experience of small babies and have read about the importance of bonding are anxious that they will not be able to respond with appropriate emotions, and that those present will criticize them for their inability to bond. In fact, for any mother there is often a phase of stunned astonishment, an interval when she needs time to find herself again. Moira expressed this when she said:

The head oozed out and then the shoulders were eased through. He came resembling a wee lizard. All my emotions were frozen in a void with this beautiful yet very ugly creature lying on my tummy. They told us how clever we were, which gave the moment warm snowflakes.

The first-time mother, whatever her age, is often rather frightened of her child initially. 'I thought she was lovely,' one woman said, 'but was scared and lived in a fog of worry and uncertainty until she was six weeks old. Then the fog cleared and miraculously there we were, the three of us intact.'

Jan was right, of course, when she suspected that the change that takes place is at least partly biological. The woman at term is primed physiologically and psychologically in readiness for motherhood. The release of hormones into her bloodstream at the time of labour is linked with uterine contractions, working to open the cervix and press the baby down the birth canal. The same hormonal surge subsequently contracts the uterus to expel the placenta and mould it back into its former shape, and drive the woman forward emotionally into motherhood. She is carried on a wave of powerful emotions, a passion that is for many women intensely sexual in its pain and pleasure. Dr Michel Odent describes oxytocin as the 'happiness hormone', released only when a woman feels she can trust herself and her body. This and other hormones flood her bloodstream during the days following birth, making her emotionally labile, vulnerable and, above all, responsible.

This acute physiological link with the baby lasts for many women for about six weeks, and for some it is much longer. It corresponds to the period of 'primary maternal preoccupation' described by Donald Winnicott, though the term does nothing to convey the powerful 'gut feelings' and the almost animal nature of the bond between the mother and her newborn. It has clearly been important to the survival of the species.

Giving – and receiving

The new mother is often enormously surprised to discover a capacity for selfless giving and patience far beyond her expectations. She is in partnership with her baby, sending out signals involving touch, scent, the rhythm of her breathing and heartbeats, her eyes turned towards the baby, and her voice raised to a higher than usual pitch, as she speaks in a pattern of five- to fifteen-second intervals, and quite unconsciously repeats the phrases with their strong beat which have meaning for all babies and in all languages.

Apparently casual, random behaviour is, in fact, perfectly adjusted to the needs and attention span of this new baby. The mother leans forward so that she is face-to-face with her baby and about a forearm's length away, the distance at which the child can most easily focus on her shining eyes and mobile mouth, and one at which it is naturally held when breastfeeding. She raises her eyebrows quite spontaneously and begins to talk. The baby's attention is caught by the movement. She smiles and the relief planes of her face are increased. In a questioning tone of voice, reiterating simple syllables, she starts to 'rev up' the baby, exaggerating her facial expression, perhaps grimacing, and may do that over and over again, like an angler throwing a line. At last the baby catches on and gets excited. Eyes light up, the lips form a shape, there may even be a little gurgle or coo of pleasure. The relationship between mother and baby is a going concern!

Far from being a passive little bundle, the newborn baby seeks stimulus, explores, and starts out on a new adventure. The child too is sending out signals and plays an active role in this partnership. She gazes at her mother's forehead, who then hovers nearer, trying to catch her eyes. Then she gets her attention and, in the early days for a brief time only, the two begin a conversation together, until the baby gets bored with it and attention wanders. The anxious mother continues to hover and try to stimulate the baby to respond. A relaxed mother releases the baby to turn to something else of interest, or to be fairly passive until the next burst of conversation between them. It is as if the two are learning a dance together. When the mother is anxious or depressed, or the baby is suffering the effect of pain-relieving drugs taken into her bloodstream during labour, or has a headache from a difficult birth, it takes longer for them to learn that dance of interaction. But it is astonishing how many mothers and babies – even though the woman feels she had no 'maternal instincts' or has been anxious that she will be 'tied down' by a baby or that her 'mind will rot' – start to enjoy each other.

They both have the advantage of much more primitive preverbal signals than we are inclined to acknowledge in adult life. Smell is one of them. Many new mothers comment on the delicious scent of their babies. The baby, for her part, responds to the mother's smell. Dr Aidan MacFarlane has shown that even five-day-old babies prefer a breastpad that has been against their own mother's breast to one worn by a strange mother. The maternal scent is intensified by heat produced in her breasts as she responds to her baby's cry. It is not only the smell of milk, but a scent emanating from her skin, that the baby senses. This is partly because the woman who has recently delivered is very warm, and during the first days after birth perspires freely, losing the fluid that was retained in her tissues in the last weeks of pregnancy. I do not know of anything that has ever been written about the smell of puerperal blood. We usually treat it as merely a messy waste-product, an aftermath of childbirth. But it has a strong, clinging and exciting smell which is in some ways intensely sexual. The baby cannot fail to be aware of this after-birth blood scent. As the baby sucks at the breast, oxytocin makes the uterus contract further and more blood is squeezed out, sometimes (especially early in the morning after lying down for some hours) in heavy, velvet clots.

For a woman who has not yet had her baby this may seem revolting. But with birth come strange, new pleasures, deep below the ground of our conscious being.

Eager to learn

At the same time a good deal of more obvious conscious cerebral activity is taking place. If you watch carefully you see that the baby is eager and quick to learn. Wait till she is in a quiet, alert state, comfortable with her body, not hungry, but wide awake and staring at you. Then stick out your tongue. The chances are that after a few false starts there will be a flicker of movement from the baby's mouth and she, too, will try to put out her tongue. After a few days, when the baby is

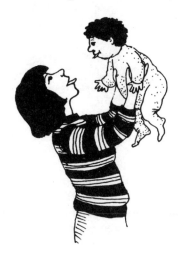

Then stick out your tongue . . .

happy and attentive, she will mimic you effectively. It is the beginning of a great game. It is on such copying that the learning of language and the general acquisition of culture is based in each society. Long before speech, the patterns of mouth movements and even facial expressions are already set.

It is important to let the baby set the pace. The over-stimulated baby, entertained too vigorously by an adult who wants to prove that he or she can be successful, turns away and gazes hard at something else, ignoring the brash stimulus and making the intruder feel rejected. If this happens, often a parent can feel a failure. Some babies enjoy more stimulus than others, so you need to get to know your baby. If you act according to the book, or set an educational scheme going that is insensitive to what your baby is telling you, the relationship is hampered from the start.

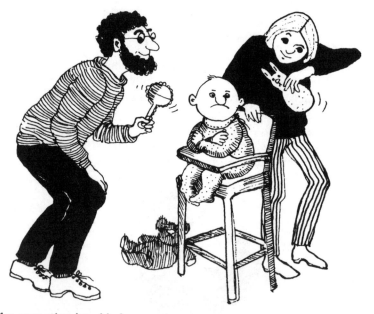

The over-stimulated baby

While the trigger for all this is a biological one important in creating the bonds of family and the handing on of culture in all human communities, the specific scene is that offered by the environment in which the mother first meets and begins to get to know her baby. For most women in the Western world nowadays, this is a hospital ward. The atmosphere provided in that setting can help or inhibit bonding.

This is only indirectly created by curtains or furnishings. It is made by *people*.

The way the relationship starts is not entirely dependent on what is happening during the time following delivery. It is in part an outcome of everything that has happened to the mother in labour and while she was pregnant. She is not merely a container for the foetus. What she feels about the act of birth and the care she is given, the way she is treated as a person, not just a caretaker for the baby, affects her ability to relate to her child. When she feels cherished and among friends, free to act spontaneously, without stopping to wonder whether she is doing the right thing, obeying the rules or reaching a set standard, she can most enjoy her baby.

With loving emotional support and in a relaxed atmosphere the most unlikely woman starts out on motherhood with gusto. It is not a matter of doing the 'right' thing; there is no right way to look after a baby. It is more a matter of doing what you feel like doing and not getting self-conscious about it. Even if you do not get the chance to be yourself while still in hospital and fall in love with your baby only after you come home, you need not feel that you have missed a limited opportunity. In human relationships there are, fortunately, second, third and even fourth chances. Each of the anxious pregnant women who were discussing with me their fears of the future and their loss of self-esteem discovered that they were surprised at the pleasure they found in what one called 'the exquisite beauty of captivity to a baby'.

A support network

If you are expecting your first baby after 35 it is a good idea to contact other women in the same age group who are having, or have just had, their babies. Your childbirth teacher or local childbirth group can put you in touch. It is helpful to have a support network afterwards, and to know that there is someone you can phone who is facing similar difficulties. Some childbirth organizations have postnatal support groups. You can either use the existing structure or get something going yourself that is specifically for older first-time mothers. One woman said:

> I got depressed. The baby was demanding and cried a lot, and I felt I'd put myself back 16 years to when I had my first baby in my teens. Then I found a drop-in playgroup and I felt part of a community of women. I booked into the postnatal network, too. They are coffee mornings, yes, but quite different from other coffee mornings. They're fantastically valuable.

It can take courage to make new contacts after the baby is born and be difficult to get out to meet people unless you have arranged things in advance. A new mother of 40, whose friends all had children in their teens, said it was a totally alien world to her and it was not till she started taking her child to playgroup that she caught up with social contacts that otherwise would have passed her by:

> I meet these efficient 20- to 25-year-olds wisely discussing child management and nursery groups. For all my grey hairs I think it must be good to have this link with a much younger group. Perhaps it will keep me feeling younger, if I'm not worn out by the effort.

Ella went through a difficult time when her daughter Penny was three to six months old, when the novelty of a baby had worn off, and when many women find endlessly repeated tasks are beginning to get them down. With Ella it was particularly hard because Penny was awake most of the day, sleeping only for half-hour stretches:

> Unlike what the books say she was definitely not happy sitting in her bouncing chair and watching Mummy doing things. *She* wanted to be doing things and found it very frustrating that she couldn't. She therefore wanted my constant attention so we could 'do' things together.

Ella felt she was 'floundering in a sea of baby and wondering if I'd ever surface'. She started shouting at her, and was then submerged in guilt. Her partner could not help as he was producing a new film and came home emotionally and physically drained late each evening. She began to feel very lonely and longing for adult company:

> I met a mother who was part of the local National Childbirth Trust (NCT) postnatal support group. From then on I never looked back. I became involved with other mothers of similar interests and backgrounds (in their thirties, had careers, etc.). I had people to share my new experiences and difficulties with and we gave each other support.

She began to help other mothers who were still at a stage through which she had passed and says this gave her 'a tremendous feeling of being of use to others apart from my baby'. Through working with this postnatal support group, Ella weaned herself from the state of total immersion in her baby. It is this period that can be so long drawn out and painful for a socially isolated mother.

Feeling tired

Your only chance of catching up on sleep may be to allow yourself to drift off when the baby sleeps during the day (all babies sleep *sometimes*). It is difficult to do this when people expect you to be up and about, the phone is ringing, and there is noise outside. But a late morning or early afternoon siesta can refresh and rejuvenate. Some people can drop off to sleep for ten minutes and wake refreshed, but for many this is worse than not going to sleep at all. A normal sleep cycle lasts 90 minutes, so this is the length for a siesta, if you can get it. But the quality as well as the length of sleep is important. To sink into a deep sleep, it helps to be in a darkened room, perhaps with music as a screen against other intrusive sound. Though it may take superhuman efforts to make this space in your life, it may be the only weapon that an older mother can seize against the fatigue that many experience, especially in the early days.

Some women need more than this – complete seclusion with the baby, taking naps whenever the baby lets them, and – for a time at any rate – screening out the external world.

One woman said that both she and her husband were 'terrified': 'Having had no contact with infants, we relied on books. I put myself into voluntary purdah, determined not to surface until I had established my confidence.'

Her relationship with her partner was strengthened by it: 'Sharing care of Gemma has been the longest sole period of shared activity in our 13 years.' On the other hand, many of those mothers who write within two years of a child's birth say that libido is much reduced, they are too exhausted for sex, and make love much less frequently than before conception.

One woman, whose youngest child is now five, says, 'The baby was so demanding and I was so tired I am surprised that the marriage survived at all sometimes.' She says she had 'nothing left over' for her husband, 'nothing left to give'. The first 18 months were 'a dark, black patch' in her life. Once this period is over, most couples seem to rediscover their sex lives.

The loss of personal time – in which *you* can decide what you want to do, or simply do nothing – comes as a shock. A 38-year-old woman with a 20-month-old and a new baby says:

My personal time is now my time with the baby, when Matt takes the older one out. I miss freewheeling brain time. There is a constant tension of having to plan ahead. I look at my friends with babies and realize that men rarely plan ahead. Women have to do it – checking the contents of the changing bag when they go out, deciding the time when you can go out – always looking ahead.

At 45, with children of 20, 18, 14 and just ten weeks, Diana's family now spreads across three generations and she says that the birth has 'thrilled and rejuvenated' her. She claims that:

> The adventure of producing and supporting this new personality is more interesting than the alternatives of middle-age career, more holidays, and outings. Our new arrival has come at an age when many of our friends are tired, bored, frustrated, and wondering what to do with themselves!

The experience has made life richer for this couple, and they feel much younger.

It is obvious that it is not just a question of learning new and difficult technical tasks. For any woman who has been until then engaged in work that has a beginning, middle and end, caring for a baby poses an entirely new activity that is never finished and that she can never assess completely. As one put it:

> I find it difficult with young children to work at full stretch with my attention divided in several different directions at once. Having been exhorted at school to 'keep your eye on the ball' and 'concentrate on the job in hand', nothing had prepared me for this.

Another, listing the things she has learned since she had her baby, says they are:

1 Rarely finishing a conversation.
2 Never eating a meal leisurely.
3 Drinking cold tea and coffee.
4 Getting jobs done while the baby is asleep.

All this makes her feel that external events are 'manipulating' her. It is sometimes made more acute for the woman who has her first baby in her late thirties because of what one calls 'a heightened awareness of problems and perhaps taking the whole experience more seriously, as a commitment and responsibility'. This, rather than simply a failure in resilience or lack of physical energy, proves most tiring. Many women say they go on in faith, not really knowing whether they are doing well or badly. There are a million and one tasks, repetitive and mundane, none of which are rewarded and most of which go unnoticed by anybody, but these are only incidental to the main activity that is completely amorphous and that continues day and night. To have to face this alone and without the support of a loving partner can be a nightmare.

Yet having a partner and other family members involved does not necessarily make it any simpler. For though it is possible to draw sustenance from their concern and caring, the birth entails radical changes being worked through and new understanding sought, and this can be a painful process. Tiredness and confusion may mean that communication breaks down and that the person who is trying most to help proves the most irritating. The birth of a child in an already formed family, or to a couple who have been together some time and have worked out a *modus vivendi* for just the two of them, compels adjustment to a network of relationships. People caught up in this begin to see themselves and each other in a new light. It can be a major growth experience in middle age.

Going back to work

Juggling a career and a baby is exciting, but it is also a gamble. It is not just a question of whether you can slot the baby into spaces in your working day or somehow compress the work so that you make gaps. You need to face the fact that your priorities may change; a new mother may realize that, after all, she cannot bear to leave her baby and that the last thing she wants to do is to hand it over to somebody else. 'I fell in love with my baby,' Jenny said. 'For the first year I didn't want to concentrate or spend time on anything or anybody else for more than a couple of hours.'

Some employers have strict rules about maternity leave. Others are open to negotiation. Olivia returned at the earliest opportunity and, 11 weeks after the birth, was longing to 'get back to the daily stimulus' of the publishers where she worked. 'I never switched on to motherhood,' she explained. Gail returned at six and a half months and felt it was too early for her. Part-time work may be the answer for you. But it has a tendency to slip into three-quarter time. Some women feel guilty about not doing 'their share' and stay longer in the office, so might just as well be working full time.

It helps to have the sort of work where you can be flexible about time or do some work at home. Or there may be the opportunity of job sharing.

It may also help if you can work near enough to home to pop back for lunch and have some time with the baby. Or you may need quiet time by yourself which is eroded if you commit yourself to that. Olivia says that her lunch hour is the only space in the 24 hours she has for herself and it is important to keep it her own. Only *you* can know what is right for you.

It is not just a matter of how you feel or what employers require, either. There is the little matter of the baby's personality, too. Some babies are easy to fit neatly into your plan. Other just do not co-operate. It was like that for Lisa:

> I planned to go back to work three months after, but Emma cried on average four hours a day and only I could comfort her. I was breastfeeding and she did so enjoy sucking, sleeping a bit, then sucking again. People said, 'Don't let the baby take over your life' and I struggled not to let that happen. But I also felt that she wouldn't be a baby for long and now was the time when I could give her what she wanted. She was like that till four and a half months and then suddenly changed and became the happiest baby imaginable. I'm glad I put off going back to work.

Anna, whose baby is four months old, is already back in full stride as a TV producer. She tries to trim her work commitments to the baby's needs, but says:

> I enjoy being a mother more than I had ever imagined and can't wait to get back to the baby. Every time I am away from her I realize I am missing new things she does, a phase of her develop-ment that will never happen again.

There are other women who want to get back to work because they find that being at home with a baby is a lonely and depressing experience. They feel cut off from adult society, isolated within four walls as they try to cope with a never-ending succession of feeds and nappy changes stretching through the 24 hours. And of course many women have to return to work because they need the money.

Before the baby is born it is difficult to work out with any accuracy exactly how it is going to be for you, either emotionally or in terms of the practical arrangements that work best. Having a baby means jumping in at the deep end, determined to do it somehow but, above all, knowing how to be flexible so that you can adapt to whatever sur-prises and challenges life presents.

In the developing world women have traditionally returned to work with the baby in a shawl straddling their hips or cocooned against their breasts or backs. Or they go to work in the fields or sell produce in the market, leaving the baby with sisters-in-law, co-wives or members of their own family – knowing that the child will be cared for in exactly the way they would themselves. In the West, patterns of childcare change so radically between generations, theories taking over from practical common sense, that a child may be pitched between completely different kinds of care-giving and divergent child-raising theories. And if a woman wants to take her baby with her to work she soon comes up against the fact that our society is not organized for mothers with small children in tow. She runs an obstacle race, sometimes with barrier after barrier put in her way.

When I was working for the Open University on a project to produce new courses on birth and babies, a notice appeared instructing staff not to bring their children into the office. In Swedish universities, in contrast, I have seen mothers – fathers too – study and teach with babies in carriers against their bodies. And crèches are provided in places of employment as a matter of course. It may be a long haul, but perhaps one of the first things a woman ought to do when she is thinking of starting a pregnancy is to get together with others to campaign for a crèche. One woman I know, reckoning that it would take between two and three years to win the battle, carefully planned her pregnancy to start two and a half years after the initiation of the campaign. The crèche was opened just in time for her to make use of it.

In the USA there is a swing away from approval of working mothers towards a heavy emphasis on the joys of motherhood and an uninterrupted relationship between mother and child. Children's books on the market include *The Terrible Thing That Happened at My House* (i.e. 'my mom went back to work'), *Just My Luck* and *Sonia's Mommy Works* – about the psychological impact of having a mother with a job. 'I wish you didn't work in an office,' says one fictional child, 'I like you at home better. That way I can tell you things and hug you.' And another complains, 'My mother used to be a real mother. But then something terrible happened to change all that and everything began to be different.' The ideal mother is firmly planted in the home, drawing complete emotional fulfilment from the love that flows between her and her children. She sits there like an angel with all-enveloping wings, a secret smile of satisfaction on her lips, glowing with tenderness, her cherubim nestled about her like cygnets beneath the mother swan. There must be few women who can live up to that image of unfailing love. It is a dangerous one because it implies that women who are not perfectly contented are complete failures as mothers. It makes a mockery of all the real *gut* feelings that come with being a mother, emotions much more powerful than the ad-man's image of motherhood ever hints at.

A working mother who hands her child over to be cared for by somebody else often has to cope with intense feelings of guilt – sometimes, too, with a good deal of anxiety as to whether she can really trust the people who are looking after her baby.

It is tricky to be a working mother not only because you have to cope with other people's attitudes to the way you split your life between work and the child, but because these doubts and fears, these feelings that you are not living up to some standard of motherhood, are inside *ourselves* too.

A working woman knows that she has to do her job better than a man and also feels that she must show that she is a 100 per cent 'good mother'. The social pressures are enormous. Lydia, a merchant banker, says: 'I have to perform better than men. And I can't take time off, as they do sometimes – for sports days and so on – to be with my children.' The emotional pressures are insidious. One woman who disliked her work and who had a steady succession of nannies was severely depressed – and her child suffered emotionally, too. His nanny was keen on potty training him when he was two: 'He used to have nightmares and screamed "potty" in his sleep.' By the time he was three he was having attacks of asthma. This mother went through a long drawn-out agony moving 'like a zombie' between work she hated and a home from which she felt outcast, deeply threatened by the nannies who took over her child. 'I would have given anything to have stayed at home,' she says, 'but we needed the money. I cannot imagine why women do it from choice.'

Finding the right person to look after your baby is basic to the whole strategy. Judy, who is a university lecturer, says that she decided personality was more important than qualifications and, though she had the chance of appointing an NNEB-trained nanny, she let her feelings guide her and chose someone she felt she would enjoy having living with them.

Jenny is in publishing and when her first marvellous nanny left after 15 months she said it 'seemed like World War III'. She advertised, discovered that many young women were only coming for interview practice and liked chopping and changing between jobs very quickly, but at last she found the right person, who has been with them now for three and a half years. She says:

> It's almost like being married to two people – your husband and your nanny. There is a lot of tension in those relationships if either thinks they are not getting your attention. When I come in through the front door I know that my husband sometimes thinks, 'Why doesn't she come and talk to me first?' It's not only that I need to find out when the last nappy change was; I can't

just treat her as an object. I can't take over from her without first being interested in how she spent her day and how things went. If anyone is living in your house like that, you have to make sure they are nurtured.

Another vital element in any effective strategy for a working mother is to have a partner, or somebody else, who is equally involved and committed to making arrangements work. This person needs to be able to give a good deal of energy, rather than drawing your energy away to meet his own needs. Single mothers, even though they have the daunting challenge of total responsibility, do not have to face the problem of a man who wants to be treated like a child himself or who is jealous of the attention the baby is getting. 'You are all three,' says Jenny, 'the mother, the father and nanny, directors on a Board of Directors called Baby Incorporated.'

Difficulties can arise when you have to rely on help where the child-carer is not sharing in decision-making in that way and is merely at the receiving end of instructions. There is often then a fight over the possession of the child, or the carer fades from the scene when you most need her. This can happen if you are relying on a relative or a minder who is only taking in children because she needs the money. The system seems to work best when the minder is someone who is, or might be, a friend of yours and has an approximately similar lifestyle.

Zoe told me that she would never have got pregnant in the first place except that her mother-in-law, 'who is potty about babies', said that she would look after the baby:

> But when I was six months' pregnant she suddenly decided not to retire after all. I was completely and utterly thrown. She didn't understand at all and said things like, 'Couldn't you make jam and sell it on a stall?' She wasn't aware that it was a terrible blow. But she did have him from four to nine months and that gave me time. A doting relative is an easy way to start. And she was very keen to do things the way I wanted. His routine was exactly the same as at home.

By the time her mother-in-law went back to work Zoe had been able to find a baby minder who was an ex-teacher with a small child herself and lived a short way up the road. 'She was marvellous,' Zoe says, 'though we had a break of a year when she had her second baby. You just cannot rely on having one good person throughout. And once your routine is thrown everything goes out of the window.'

Some working mothers find that sharing a nanny is the best solution. The nanny is employed by one family and a few other children come each day. It often does not work if there are more than three children as it is difficult for the nanny to get out with them. If she is stuck in the house all day she may feel trapped and resentful. And the children may lack the stimulus they would get if they went to mother and toddler groups.

A head teacher told me that she felt the share-a-nanny scheme often put a great strain on the children. Three- and four-year-olds are literally banned from their own homes and get very over-tired while they wait for Mummy to finish evening surgery or to get back from her office. And some of the mothers pointed out that there can be friction because the nanny shows favouritism towards her own charges, or other people's kids seem to make more mess than your own, eat more food, and use up more electricity.

There can be other problems with nannies, whether they are your own or you are sharing them with another family too. Some, according to one mother I talked to, are 'very snobby. We were not good enough. She liked to have children whose parents "were something".' Another said that she found her nanny competitive, vying with others to demonstrate how advanced or well-behaved her charges were.

No system seems to work well for everybody and it is important to shop around in advance to find what is available. Continuity of care is essential if small children are to have a sense of security – and for your own peace of mind. 'If I thought my children were being passed from one person to another,' one mother, who is a senior civil servant, said, 'that would finish me.'

It is possible to continue breastfeeding and work outside the home, but that too needs planning ahead. Sally is an administrator with a rail company and had not managed to get her baby on to the bottle when she had to go back to work: 'I was nearly demented. He wouldn't take a bottle and he wasn't interested in solids. Then I got blocked milk ducts.'

If you know you are going back to work it makes sense to get a small hand pump and express some milk, which someone else can then give to the baby in a bottle. You need to start this before the baby is about four months old to be sure that she will take it. It is often possible to give a couple of morning feeds before going to work, and then two, or even three, in the evening. That way, you keep up your supply of breastmilk.

Nicky takes a pump to the office and expresses each lunchtime, storing it in the office fridge before taking it home to be used the following day. This means she does not get uncomfortable with her breasts swollen and throbbing in the afternoon. It ensures that she has enough milk. For breasts need stimulus if they are to go on supplying milk, and if you go a long time between feeds expressing helps provide that stimulus.

Breastmilk stores well for 24 hours at ordinary fridge temperature. You can also freeze it if you want to. Some mothers are happy to have a night-waking baby because a night feed then makes up for one missed during the day. Others are only too glad to drop night feeds as soon as possible or prefer to give the baby a bottle at night if they have a partner willing to do it. Either way, a baby can still have breastmilk if you learn how to use a pump and, if necessary, experiment with different kinds until you find one that is right for you. The Breastfeeding Promotion Group of the National Childbirth Trust is always willing to help.[5]

In spite of all the difficulties and the sheer wizardry that is often needed to combine work and motherhood so that you enjoy both, many women say they would not have it any other way. Jill, who is a town planner, says that going back to work was the most difficult decision she ever had to make: 'But I came to the conclusion that I need to achieve something. I wanted a break from my child to do something which was me – and to keep me sane!' She comes back from work to take pleasure in her child in a way that she feels she never could if she was around all the time. Cheryl, a teacher, says she enjoys the lovely quiet weekends with her baby. They both have a very active time during the week, she at a sixth form college and her two-year-old's nanny steers him through a 'wild social life with other children' so that they relish being quiet together on the other two days.

There are other benefits, too. If you and your partner have normally lived fairly independent and equal lives, each with your own income, and sharing housework and cooking, it can be important for you to retain that independence after you have a baby. An architect told me:

> I didn't do it just for myself. I really thought it was vital for our relationship as a couple that I went back to work. We've had children late and I would be very frustrated and hell to live with if I couldn't go on being independent.

Another bonus is that parenthood is an education and you development management skills of which you never realized you were capable. One woman with a full-time job told me that now she is packing far more into her life and that this in itself is satisfying: 'I know I have a limited amount of time and I am much better organized since I had a child.' She reckons that these management skills make almost any woman who is combining motherhood and a job qualified for an immediate directorship!

7

Partners

Babies thrive when they are cared for by more than one loving adult. This simple fact, reflecting the kind of cherishing in the family that babies receive all over the world, has been obscured by psychological pronouncements on the part of experts who have threatened mothers with causing incalculable damage to their infants if they do not commit themselves to full-time mothering day in, day out, for the first three years of the child's life.

The power of John Bowlby's work[1] to grip women with fear that they were neglecting and depriving their children when they handed over to another adult for a well-earned break affected a whole generation of mothers, and often made them feel resentful of the baby who was trapping them within four walls, and guilty that they felt the resentment. It was not, of course, Dr Bowlby's fault. His research was caught up in an insidious social force that in the 1960s was driving women back to the

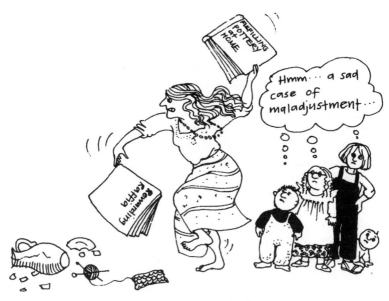

Women ought to find their fulfilment in the home . . .

111

home to be good wives and mothers and telling them that they ought to find all their fulfilment there. If you could not, you were not a 'real' woman. Mothers reared children, collected cotton reels and empty cartons, baked bread, and cultivated the home arts as if their lives depended on it. We thought we were doing our best for our children. Some struggled to do things outside the home as well, but without our husbands or children noticing.

Indoctrinating a mother with the notion that she is the one person who matters in her child's life is an element in the suppression of women as potential wage-earners and creators outside the purely domestic sphere. Domestic work has always been second class.

It is easy for a mother to make herself essential to a small child, easy to build such an intense one-to-one relationship, with no room for any other adult's participation, such that the child cannot be left with anyone else, will not accept comfort from them, and suffers acute trauma of separation if she attempts to cut the bond. The woman whose only emotional rewards are in her family may make herself indispensable to her children because otherwise she is nothing.

In societies in which other family members and friends and neighbours share care of small children the child moves easily from one to the other. Of course she knows who her mother is, even if the compound is shared with co-wives and their children, but the relationship is not so exclusive that it rules out other attachments. The mother–child tie is one of a whole pattern of rich relationships. Among the Ganda, Schaffer and Emerson[2] found that by the time babies were 18 months old all but a handful of children were emotionally attached to more than one person, and often to several. The father was most likely to be the chief of these attachment figures. But toddlers were also attached to older children who acted as care-givers.

There is a very special time in the life of any mother and baby when the relationship is intense in a different way, which I touched on earlier. This is during the first six to eight weeks of the child's life, the period that Donald Winnicott called that of 'primary maternal preoccupation', when the psycho-physiological bond of a lactating mother to her infant is often so strong that it pre-empts other relationships, seems to blot out the rest of the world, and causes her to respond to and protect her baby like a tigress defending her young. 'I had never realized before,' one woman said, 'how much I was an animal – gloriously so.' Some women say that this affects all their emotions, which become more concentrated and are experienced more passionately.

A primitive bond

This phase of new motherhood is so distinct that anybody else behaving in such a way would be considered pathologically disturbed. Yet it is a natural part of being a mother. It is the recognition of this primitive bond between mother and neonate that has in some ways been allowed to spill over into the whole of the rest of motherhood, and is sometimes accepted as the norm for women with ten-month-old babies, and two-year-old and four-year old and eight-year old children. When the mother cannot function in this emotional intensity, or feels crushed by the demands made on her, she believes there must be something wrong with her.

The woman starting out on motherhood in her thirties or forties for the first time is often rather afraid of this. She has watched other women with babies, and from the vantage point of her career has seen what has happened to fellow students and colleagues. This may be one reason why she has put off having a child. She wanted freedom to live her own life first, to put her education to some use, to achieve something. As one put it, 'I needed to protect my individuality.' Another said, 'I feel I was conditioned by what everyone else wanted to do or has done. I needed to free myself to think out what I wanted to do and make it my own decision.' And yet another expressed it in this way:

I was an independent, ambitious career woman with a happy marriage based on the principle of equality. I regard this stage of motherhood (with little ones) as temporary and a temporary pause in my career development. I imagine I will return to my former dynamic, individual, ambitious self. If I had had a baby in my twenties I would have found motherhood claustrophobic, crippling my independence and freedom. I couldn't even consider marriage then, so strong was my desire to be free.

This woman is sometimes aware that in a way she 'mothers' her partner and is anxious lest the baby's claims for attentions compete with his. It is important for them to discuss such anxieties in advance of the birth. A good childbirth class in which there is plenty of free discussion and sharing between expectant parents lets them do just that, and discover that other couples have the same doubts and apprehensions. Penny and Leo have been together for five years. His mother left him as a baby and he was brought up by his father. Penny said she knew she mothered him:

That side is strong in our relationship. Sometimes he says, 'I won't be your baby any more.' Oh! That sounds soppy! He feels threatened by the baby. But I have seen him with small babies and he's lovely with them. I've tried to reassure him.

Prue comments on what Penny is saying:

I feel the same with my husband. It was my decision to have the baby and there was no encouragement. But I've seen him with children. He's changed a lot with the pregnancy. First of all he wasn't interested at all. He was worried and said, 'I don't feel old enough to have a family.' He didn't want to be tied down. Now he's looking forward to it – he's totally changed.

Lyn says:

When I first realized I was pregnant, Dick's attitude was, 'Oh God!' He used to treat children like Martians, incomprehensible! He stood back from them. Now I've noticed him seeming more relaxed, not just with children, but a kind of emotional freedom. He used to be very self-contained emotionally. The pregnancy had given a legitimate channel for feelings that have been kept out and that he has never experienced before. This has had a very positive effect on our relationship.

The dynamics of psychological change when a couple share together the emotional as well as physical preparation for a baby are such that each is better able to meet the stresses that come after and enjoy the inevitable change in their relationship. As one woman said, it was not only that they were very happy about the pregnancy, it was also a 'bonding' of two people.

Shared responsibility

A loving partner who shares parenting with an equal sense of responsibility is the foundation of life for those women who describe themselves as happy and confident mothers. One woman looking back 18 years later to the birth of her twins at 35, and the subsequent experience of parenting with a husband who she says, 'took a full share in caring for the children from the start', comments:

We have discovered ourselves. There is a whole area of one's character that emerges in parenthood, in the way one copes . . . and in communicating with one's children. This has been a continuing surprise over the years.

This partner is often a husband, sometimes a lover, sometimes another woman, but the woman alone without anyone to share parenting, or who struggles to bring up a child while her partner is immersed in career and success outside the home, is invariably at a disadvantage. The majority of women who wrote made explicit statements about ways in which they worked out together their joint commitment as parents. A woman having her first baby at this age who has worked outside the home over a period of some years, together sharing household chores in an egalitarian way, is more likely to plan a strategy of this kind with her partner than women who already have families and who go on to have another baby or start another family after an interval, sometimes with a new husband. It is the middle-aged second husband who tends to see his main responsibilities as outside the home and to leave childcare exclusively to his wife.

But for any man who feels under pressure at work and is climbing a career ladder, home tends to be 'off duty' time when peace and quiet, contentment and some conviviality are expected. He feels under heavy financial responsibility and looks on it as a place of relaxation where he can enjoy an interval with his wife and child. These are the fathers who play with their children and sometimes 'help', but who feel no responsibility for childcare. Some of these women who are left 'holding the baby' sound a note of regret and some obviously feel trapped in their roles as mothers, at least for the time being, and are critical of the absent partner.

Olivia had one child at 27 and her second at 36 after being told by her gynaecologist that she would not be able to have any more children, and failing to adopt. Laurence is a university lecturer. Olivia says that he helped much more with the first baby because:

He was very jealous of my ability to feed him and wanted to do everything for him that he could. This time Laurence isn't at home as much. His job is very demanding and time consuming and he travels away from home frequently. He has perhaps changed the baby's nappy once a week if I'm lucky. Our roles have become more 'typed' than ten years ago. Laurence's work has very high priority for all of us. We don't have the equality of job prospects that we shared in our early twenties.

Una is 40, with children aged 13, 11, and 9, and before the birth of the new baby she was a part-time college lecturer. Her husband has long days in the office and gets home late, so does not help with domestic work or the children. Una says:

I wonder whether I shall ever be able to get a job now, my age and

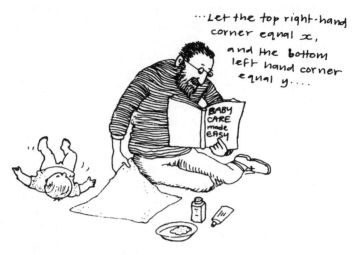

...Let the top right-hand
corner equal x,
and the bottom
left hand corner
equal y....

Laurence is a university lecturer . . .

the numbers of unemployed increasing together. I have pangs of jealousy at my husband's career success as I was once just as brainy and well qualified as he was. What really bugs me is that if he wants a regular evening out he can have one. If I want a regular evening out he says I can have one, but then has to be away with his job.

She confesses that she feels intellectually frustrated and resentful.

Teresa has just had her second baby after postnatal depression for a year following her first child's birth. He is now two and a half and it is clear from the way she writes that puerperal hormone changes give a very inadequate explanation for the depression into which she is sinking again. He husband was 'thrilled' with the pregnancy but, she says:

I'd have appreciated help with shopping and heavy housework. I deeply resented him for not offering, after I'd said a couple of times I needed help, and I was too proud to go on asking. He thinks of fatherhood as having a 'nice cuddle' and playing with 'pretty, well-cared-for kids' but should also have the experience of disposing of the daily piles of grubby clothes and dirty nappies, planning and cooking balanced meals and shopping for them and tidying up toys. He's very good at entertaining David for hours but leaves a stream of toys, books, used cups and clothes in his wake, which are apparently invisible to him once they have served their purpose. If I go out it doesn't occur to him to plan and produce a meal for the child.

She worked full time till David was nine months old, a very stressful period because she felt torn between the child and her work, and total responsibility for him and running of the home fell on her. 'When David was ill it was always me who took time off work. Men have a long way to go,' she concludes, 'before they are truly fathers the way women are mothers to their children.'

Conditioned mothers

It is not just that men often take it for granted that women are responsible for baby care and domestic work and expect them to be better at looking after babies than they are, women themselves are socially conditioned to feel *they* ought to be home-makers and child rearers to such an extent that a mother may shut the father out of full participation in parenting. Jill, aged 36 and doing part-time teaching, cannot help herself because the emotions are so strong. She feels depressed, tired and 'in a state of confusion about my roles of mother/wife/worker', and weighed down by 'a terrible responsibility'. She added:

> Even though I trust my husband when he is dealing with Sean I feel that I am on duty. I hover and remind him of things. He would rather be left to get on with it! Our relationship as a couple has been very much affected. I have become aware that at times I exclude Mike in my baby-centred world . . . we are like ships passing in a fog.

The marriages of some mothers who wrote had already broken up under this kind of strain. Hannah, for instance, says that the relationship 'floundered under the stress of responsibilities which I was left to bear'. They now live on different levels of a big house. She brings up her son, but his father is 'his best play-partner and brings him many things that I cannot offer'.

The social isolation that many mothers feel with their small children is peculiar to our Western, urban society. In Muslim societies, which represent for many in the West the epitome of female subjugation, women have a vigorous and highly colourful autonomous world in their own quarters, from which men are excluded.[3] A sisterhood of women share in childcare, both in the practical tasks and emotional support of the new mother.

The Indian woman is similarly part of a group consisting of her husband's brother's wives, his mother and unmarried sisters. There is no privacy, but at the same time there is no loneliness.[4]

In the Caribbean, women are part of a sisterhood network helping, gossiping about, counselling and sharing with one another, often bemoaning their lot at the hands of men who they feel are good for nothing, and striving in common to feed their children, clothe them, get them through school and 'grow them right'. In each village, three leaders, all women, act as primary communicators between every household, the postmistress, the schoolmistress and the midwife.[5, 6] In rural areas to be isolated is impossible, and the same pattern of social organization infiltrates the life of the clusters of shack dwellings and the homes of the poor in the towns.

Women are often told that depression suffered after childbirth is the result of major hormonal changes and the distress they feel is all put down to physiological processes over which they have no control. Though this may be cheering for some, for at least it is not their 'fault', it perpetuates the misery for many women, who are thereby absolved from the responsibility or opportunity to change the social conditions in which they function from day to day as mothers, which are the real cause of their distress. It is only too easy for a man, also, to explain a woman's depression by reference to her hormones and, apart from urging her to see the doctor, do nothing else about it. If she does go to the doctor, drug treatment often does not cure her. A controlled trial of the commonly prescribed antidepressant imipramine revealed that it was no better than a placebo.[7]

To be alone in a house with total responsibility for a screaming baby who seems to be crying *at* you and telling you what a hopeless mother you are is a *social* situation that has nothing to do with whether you have a uterus and breasts. One woman said, 'I go and hide in the bathroom when she cries. Maybe I do that instead of flinging her down the stairwell.' It is not only mothers who do this. Distraught babysitters and au pairs who cannot quieten the infant do it too.

Doctors, health visitors, childbirth educators and other counsellors continue to reassure the new mother that all that is needed is a readjustment of hormones, an attitude that stems from a uterine psychology which had its origins in the Middle Ages and from concepts of hysteria as the result of a wandering womb. Freudian theory reinforced this ideology of the female mind as a direct consequence of anatomy and laid down that a woman's reproductive system was 'the site for the acting out of impulses, especially aggression, and its derivative, sex anxiety, and maternity-pregnancy fears'.[8] No such claims have been made about men's mood swings, the inference being that they are more cerebral and less chained to their physiology. Yet as Ann Oakley points out,[9] monthly cycles have been reported for men in body temperature, weight and beard growth, and pain threshold and cyclical rhythms have been discovered in emotional changes, urine levels of hormones, and schizophrenia, manic depression and epilepsy.

The father's role

In fact, it cannot be assumed that women are the only ones to experience postnatal depression. Childbirth is a major life crisis for many couples, and becoming a father can be just as stressful for a man as the transition to motherhood is for a woman. Sometimes he is so overwhelmed by his own feelings that he is unable to give the woman the emotional support she needs. As men get more involved in the experience of birth, not just as members of a supporting cast, but as full emotional participants, they encounter many of the psychological conflicts that are typical of the passage to new social roles. They experience the primary preoccupation with the baby which, until now, has been thought to be a female characteristic.

It used to be believed that men must always be strong, that they must not show their emotions, and their main task was to provide economic support, leaving all the feeling to the woman; but now things have changed. A new emotional involvement means that couples have a chance to share in being parents and be open with each other as never before. Those who experience this partnership find it an enriching and often completely unexpected bonus of parenthood.

It can be hard for a man to get involved with a baby and to bond when it has been 'produced by the hospital' as a 'specialist medical product', and he feels that the whole process of having a baby is so risky that it is best to leave it all to the 'experts'. Fathers, like mothers, also find it difficult to develop confidence in handling the baby if they feel they are second-rate care-givers and that someone is watching to see if they do it properly. There are some situations in which both parents are more likely to feel that the baby is the property of the hospital and to be very apprehensive about taking on responsibility for this precious new life. When a baby had been in special care, especially in a hospital where parent participation is not encouraged, a man may be so anxious that the simplest solution seems to get out of the house and concentrate on his own work.

In those special care units, however, where both parents are welcome at any time of the day or night and shown how they can help look after their baby, confidence develops very early on. Most of the studies that have been published about this emphasize the benefits for the mother.[10] But the effect on the father is often astonishing, and changes an understandable hesitation and fear in handling his baby to super-competence and pleasure in a matter of a few hours. The self-confidence he develops then indirectly can help the mother too and give her the emotional support she needs. It sometimes seems that the emotional energy released when a man tends to his very tiny or sick baby flows beyond the infant, and in a mysterious way enables the mother to feel cherished too. Perhaps not having to go on as if nothing has happened and keep the proverbial stiff upper lip allows him to come closer to her feelings, so that they share this difficult emotional journey with more understanding of each other's vulnerability.

Though Michael's first view of his eight-week-old premature twins in special care was, he says, 'very fearsome' because they were wired up to 'things going bleep, bleep, bop', he states that when he visited the unit after that first time he hardly noticed the apparatus, only his babies. He had to overcome apprehension about interfering with the smooth running of the unit, but quickly realized that the staff were welcoming and wanted him there: 'We were all in it together.'

One of the babies was suffering from RDS, respiratory distress syndrome, because her lungs were inadequately inflated. Their normal lining, like the bubbles in detergent, was only partially present, and as a result they collapsed between each breath and the sides stuck together like plastic bags. Then she had to make a terrific gasping effort to take the next breath.

Michael stood over her in the plastic box in which she struggled for life, helpless to do anything, until a nurse suggested that he should hold her hand. As he did so he felt not only compassion and love, but as if the baby were giving *him* comfort. He started to stroke the little arm and talk to her soothingly. 'She seemed to relax,' he said. The baby was linked to apparatus that measured the amount of oxygen in her blood. He had been shown how to read this and, to his surprise, saw that when he stimulated her in this way the oxygen content went up from about 60 to 90. After three-quarters of an hour doing this, he noticed that she liked the inside of her thigh stroked and seemed to 'feel safer'. She began to breathe more easily and he again saw the results on the oxygen meter.

Michael's relationship with his baby is a far cry from that of another father who though, his wife Janet says, is 'close' to his son, needed her encouragement to 'become involved on the physical side, changing nappies, bathing him, feeding him, etc. As with most domestic matters,' she explains, 'he'd rather not be involved', and finds it easier now that the child, who is two and a half, can communicate and is not just an object with needs. This baby was born six weeks early by Caesarean section and spent time in a special care unit which was less liberal and welcoming to parents. He developed jaundice and was taken back there again. Though she does not say how her partner feels, Janet says she felt 'intimidated' while in hospital.

Breaking down barriers

A father's relationship with his new baby affects the relationship with his partner, too. It may have been partly because Michael was so stirred by the experience with his little daughter that he could be honest about his emotions. Janet said, 'I can have a weep without him thinking I'm stupid, and if he weeps I don't think, "You're a man. You're not supposed to cry." ' They were able to support each other in a way that is impossible if a couple rely on artificial hope and cheerfulness all the time. This partnership continued after the babies were home and is a firm basis from which they cope with the household disruption and sheer hard work that twins inevitably entail.

But it is not, of course, only when things are difficult that a partner is needed. Many women write of the joy they experience when childbirth is shared and say, 'I could not have done it without him there.' They say that the man's presence during labour and his emotional surrender at delivery is profoundly moving for them and that they will never forget this time. For the newly delivered woman it is not only the sight and feeling of the newborn lying on her body, but what this means to him and his spontaneous emotional release into tears, laughter and caresses. One man just said very slowly and clearly, 'Wow . . . wooow . . . wooooow!' Not all fathers express themselves with dramatic abandon! Another, after having kissed his wife and told her how clever she was, picked up the baby and danced round the room with her, singing 'Waltzing Matilda'. Some women say that although they did not have any strong sense that the baby belonged to them following delivery, when they saw the baby held in its father's arms and *his* response to his child, there was a rush of emotion and they promptly fell in love.

Sara and Phillip decided to have their second baby at home. Phillip describes it:

It is hard, impossible, to communicate to others the joy and wonder I experienced as my son slid out of Sara and, with his mother's help, on to her breast. Dan's tongue was belting away as if he had crawled into a desert oasis and was searching for the life-sustaining nectar.

Sara handed the baby to Phillip as she delivered the placenta. He said:

For the first time the reality of this life creation that Sara and I had shared for nine months was driven home . . . The birth of one's own child is the happiest, most powerful experience a man can hope to witness.

When the midwife had gone home they slept the rest of the night with their little daughter too, all four together in the large bed. 'She was curled against me,' said Sara, 'and Dan and Phillip.'

The intensity of such an experience for both parents prepares the way for the powerful emotions that follow. Many couples say, 'We are closer.' One woman added, 'In labour I learned to trust him absolutely. When Jake was born we were so deeply moved. Somehow that deepened our understanding of each other.'

The birth is one point in an emotional journey together that involves transformations in a couple's relationship as the child grows and they discover new aspects of themselves. Sometimes these discoveries can be disconcerting and changes invariably produce fresh stresses as well as new closeness, sharpening and further defining the elements of their partnership. One man, asked how he felt the birth of their daughter, now two, had affected their relationship, said, 'It's strengthened the pluses of our marriage and deepened the minuses.'

Birth need not be a one-off, isolated emotional 'trip', though it is often reduced to that. It is part of a continuum in the relationship. Sharing in the birth of the child is a psychological experience of such significance that it gives an opportunity for them to go on from there to evolve a richer life together as caring, sharing parents as well as lovers.

8

Coping with the family

I got pregnant accidentally. When I told my 16-year-old I was pregnant, he said, 'Hah! You talk to me about sex. But what about you? It's about time you started using condoms!'

Another woman, Ann, said:

It was awkward telling the children. Eventually, at about four and a half months, after getting them together one Saturday morning, Simon asked them to guess our news. They guessed we were divorcing, separating, going abroad, that he'd been fired, but none guessed correctly. They were amazed. The boys (20 and 18) were easy-going and thought it was 'a good idea', but Susan (14) left the room and became very quiet. The next day she implied that it was thoughtless of us to let this happen.

For many couples having a second family after a gap find the most difficult people to tell are their adolescent children. It is as if the open acknowledgement of sexual activity between parents compromises the

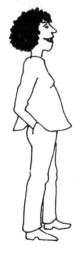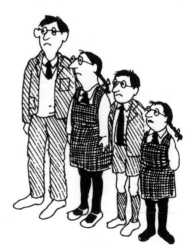

I found it awkward to tell the children

young people in their own sexual identity. Boys may be horrified, and at this age they tend to be embarrassed by having a mother who looks pregnant. Girls say, 'How could you, Mother!' as if she were discovered in some gross impropriety. One girl said to her father, 'You naughty boy, Daddy!' and he was embarrassed in turn. A boy of 11 exclaimed, 'Oh, Mum, now you've gone and done it!' He could not touch his mother right through pregnancy or, at first, touch the baby. Another seemed concerned about his mother, but only, she suggests, because he wanted to be sure she could continue to cook his dinner!

One woman, who started a second family with a new partner after a long gap, said:

> Steven, at 16, was very much against the idea of a baby. He became anxious and depressed. He was articulate about his feelings: he said it made him feel that he and Joseph were just remnants of a failed marriage. He realized that the focus of the family would shift and that the boys would no longer be the centre of attention. And both of them were worried that there would be less money – in particular that there wouldn't be enough to buy the clothes they wanted and their trainers!

Ingrid says of her 14-year-old: 'She worried about her friends' reactions to my appearance and her grades being impaired by "a screaming baby".' Another girl of this age 'went through two very traumatic years and definitely resented the intrusion of noise, demands, toys and nappies and the time consumed by a baby,' her mother says. 'Whether her adolescent years would have been so difficult without the child I don't know, but in suffering we grow as people and at nearly seventeen she has become well balanced.'

Loneliness

Even if their initial reactions are negative, older boys who have already gained confidence in their own identity often seem to cope well with the experience. But this may take time. Steven, for example, took to his bed for the first day after the birth. His mother said:

> That was terribly painful. I wanted him to see the baby while he was brand new. He was in the next room, watching TV. The midwife went in and said, 'Come on, come and see the baby!' He resented that a lot – someone outside the family interfering. When I was up and about with the baby he was averting his eyes every time we came near. Eventually I couldn't stand it any

longer, and said, 'I've got needs, too, and this hurts me. I need your help!' I started giving him the baby to hold when I was busy. I didn't make a big deal out of it, and the barriers gradually slipped down. Now the baby is two, and he has turned full circle. He decides he won't go out so that he can babysit, he carries him on his shoulders, and they go to the swings. He takes him out to meet his friends.

Girls often identify unselfconsciously with their mothers in a caring and compassionate way. A girl sometimes worries for her mother, too. One woman says that her daughter of 12 bought her nappies out of her pocket money. Frances, a single mother with a daughter of ten, who has just had another baby, says she did not realize how lonely her daughter had been before this:

She was fantastically interested. We got the Open University course and she filled in the chart and did the quizzes counting herself as my partner, read all the books and was very, very good at the relaxation exercises. She cried when I lit a cigarette or had a drink, so I stopped. She was all the things supportive partners are supposed to be. Towards the end of pregnancy she got very tense. We must have had the largest list of phone numbers and emergency procedures!

Anna feels that her pregnancy is a very good experience for her daughter of 13 and says she has 'shared' it:

I have tried to keep her in touch with all my body changes and she has seen me naked. I feel it will be a help to her in the future to have absorbed all this, rather than come to it 'cold' as I did.

However the information is received initially, most families seem to adjust not only well, but with delight, to a late addition. The 11-year-old who would not touch his mother or the baby started playing with his sister in her first year, though fairly roughly ('she loved it', his mother said), and is now 'very tender and attached'. Women say that it brings out a new-found tenderness in their sons and believe that it is a very positive preparation for later fatherhood. The 'macho' image typical of many male adolescents' picture of themselves gives way to gentleness and concern, and the whole family benefits. They no longer tear through the house with gangs of youths, and even the music may be turned down. 'Our family life has become softer and more caring,' one woman says. A 16-year-old big brother changes his baby sister's nappies and is very gentle and playful with her; 'He's mind blowing', an 18-year-old says of his newborn brother; 'terrific', a 16-year-old comments on his baby sister. An older brother of 20 remarks that he likes the changed form of the family now that it cuts right across the generations and unites them all.

After she has adjusted to the idea, an adolescent daughter may become much closer to her mother in shared womanhood, sometimes even in a kind of female conspiracy against men. One mother said of her daughter: 'She became more and more involved and helpful. She offered to stay with me for the birth, to be "a reliable help, unlike Daddy" as she put it.'

It may be important for a girl to have time with her mother alone after the birth to discuss her often very conflicting feelings. While mother and baby are in hospital this is often impossible, and after their return home there are so many visitors and such a lot of work that this time for quiet sharing can be crowded out. Elizabeth says her daughter developed a bad sore throat. They had a 'good gossip' together the first time they were alone after the birth. Elly, who had been very excited about the baby coming and involved in all the details of pregnancy, told her mother that she was worried that she did not love the baby immediately. Elizabeth said *she* felt just like that too and explained how it often took some time to get to know a baby.

Adolescents are good babysitters, though women say that they try not to make this a bind or take it for granted, and many make a regular arrangement to pay brothers and sisters for time spent doing this. A mother may find her son mending the motorbike with the baby bouncing in her seat watching the fascinating proceedings. The younger child seems to benefit greatly, though one mother says she is anxious lest the baby, present 'during the usual teenage arguments', grows up undisciplined.

Being with older children provides an intellectual stimulus for the baby, but mothers describe ways in which they make sure that the younger child is able to meet children of about the same age too. They notice how they themselves are enriched by contact with younger women and their children, opening a whole new social world, which they might not have thought they would have enjoyed in the past, but that keeps them in touch with attitudes and concerns of couples still in their twenties.

Listening to heartbeats

Children between four or five and early adolescence are rarely surprised by a pregnancy and some have been urging their mothers to have a baby for years. For girls, friends at school who have younger babies at home to look after are considered very special. The changes of pregnancy are followed with curiosity and women say that this is a great educational opportunity for their older children. Both boys and girls can listen to the baby's heartbeats through a foetal stethoscope. If you know how your baby is lying you may be able to locate the foetal heart without difficulty in the last two or three months of pregnancy.

Lie back against pillows on a couch or bed and first feel with your hands where the most actively moving small knobs are at the moment. These are probably the feet, often at one side or the other under your ribs. If the baby is active at the time, an older child can feel the kicks. Follow the legs round to the other side and you will reach the trunk; move down from there, about two hands' breadth, sliding your hand in a little as you do and you reach the spot where it is probably easiest to hear the foetal heart. You will be at tummy button level or below. If the baby has engaged in your pelvis with its head down like an egg in an eggcup, this spot will be below your umbilicus and out to the left or right side. Instead of a stethoscope you can use the cardboard cylinder from the middle of a lavatory paper roll or a tumbler with the open end placed over the area where you hope to pick up sounds. When a baby is lying with its back against your spine the limbs are at the front of your abdomen and it may be more difficult to detect the heartbeat because they are in front of its chest. If your umbilicus sinks in with a saucer-shaped depression in this area this is probably the position your baby is in at the moment. If it sticks out with a rounded shape like a water melon behind it, your baby is probably lying in the more usual anterior position and it will be easier to pick up the heartbeat. In the seventh and eighth months babies change position frequently, often many times a day, so trying another time, when the baby has shifted, may lead to success.

Women describe the wonder their older children express when they hear the baby's heartbeats or are helped to locate the different parts of the baby and feel the movements. Antenatal clinics are held during school hours, but some mothers take an older child during the holidays so that she can understand what is happening, and indirectly learn more about changes that may take place in her own body, too, in later years.

Some women choose to give birth at home partly because they feel that understanding about and sharing in birth can be important for the older children. The younger the other children, the more the mother is concerned about separation from them; the older they are, the more she sees the birth as a maturational experience for her sons and daughters.

Mary is 40, her children are aged 13, 11 and 9 – a girl and two boys. She says that after having amniocentesis she got 'hooked into the hospital system', but was unhappy about the conveyor belt atmosphere of the antenatal clinic and discovered that visiting by other siblings on postnatal wards was at weekends only. So she cancelled her booking and arranged a home birth, a really family-centred experience. When she was in the first stage of labour 'my eldest son came in and was a classic case of pacing up and down saying "Are you all right?" The midwife chatted to him and he became much more relaxed.' After the birth her daughter spent several hours just holding the baby. 'She called her several times "a dear little kitty" and I remembered that a kitten was the only pet she'd had. The feelings about the two must have been similar.'

Children can be invited to help with preparations for the new baby. This works best if they have some creative input and can use their own ideas. Sam, aged five, has fabric paints, and is painting giraffes, elephants and hedgehogs on cotton shirts.

Changing relationships

Older mothers with whom I have talked all say that though dealing with a family is hectic and exhausting, it is great fun. Lisa worried that school-age children might be ashamed that their mother was no longer youthful. She remembers how she thought her own mother was fat and dumpy and how she was torn between loyalty to her and competing with school friends who all seemed to have chic, interesting mothers. But Lisa, at 41, in jeans and T-shirt, with hennaed hair, looks much younger than her own mother, in pastel twin-set and pearls and with carefully permed hair, did at 35. And the fact that Lisa has many interests outside the home, reads widely and is mentally alert, means that she tackles bringing up children as an exciting challenge in quite a different way from her mother's style of parenting. 'The children keep me on my toes, make me stay young, I suppose,' she says. Lisa and James have changed their circle of friends, though. Most acquaintances of their own age have children at school now, and they talk about discipline, the teenage drug scene, sex education and subjects like that, whereas Lisa still finds potty-training a riveting topic! They have made new friends, much younger than they are, through the mother and toddler group and the postnatal support group with which Lisa does voluntary work. She says:

It was difficult at first. Our friends were all past this stage and it disrupted their lives to have toddlers around. Our home we'd made childproof, nothing on low tables, electric sockets stopped up, fireguards – all that sort of thing. But they'd forgotten all about that and they couldn't cope at all.

James, at 45, is a fully involved father. He does not just 'help' – he shares. When he is at home he does all the things Lisa does and is enjoying discovering new skills. Friends of his age crack mostly unfunny jokes about the zest with which he has taken to fatherhood. He does not let this worry him and says he is doing what *he* wants to do. Most days he does nappy-changing, dresses his baby daughter, washes, feeds her and plays with her. When I asked what he most liked about being a father he said: 'Having a person who is completely dependent upon you, clinging to you in complete and utter trust and faith.' For him and Lisa, the advantages of having a 'late baby' far outweigh the difficulties.

When the baby is born, new patterns of relationships in the family emerge. If a woman is preoccupied with her baby or feeling tired, older children tend to turn to their father more and also to become more self-reliant. This is very different from the more usual change in pattern when a newborn is introduced into a family where the older children are still under about five. Then an older child, the displaced baby, may regress temporarily and a typical description of the mother of a two-year-old after the birth of a new baby is:

When Dinah came to visit at the hospital she had a good look at the baby, Joe, and then got very whingeing and noisy. My husband was suffering from a hangover so each bang and clatter made him wince. When we came home she would poke Joe through the bars of his cot 'to see if he's awake'. The poor child suffered from lack of sleep for a few weeks. When I was feeding Joe she would say she wanted a wee, so I would either have to have the pot in the room with me, or try to get Dinah on the loo with Joe hanging on to his means of nourishment for grim life.

With older children the mother often gets the opposite impression – they suddenly grow up. She starts to see them through new eyes and is often astonished at the blossoming of qualities of caring and tenderness that she did not realize they possessed. One woman, commenting on the relationship of her three teenagers with their baby brother, says: 'They have all been so positive and beautiful with him this must be one of the biggest plusses of all.' And a father, summing up the effect of the birth on the older children, aged 20 down to 14, says: 'All seem to enjoy the change in structure that the baby has brought. Each child feels much more mature and responsible . . . It has given the family a focus.'

One problem with delaying a family, however, is that your parents may be ill, or may have died, at a time when you would like them to be able to enjoy (and help) with their grandchildren. Felicity is sad that her mother cannot share the excitement of her granddaughter's baby days. Right through Felicity's pregnancy she was ill, and Felicity oscillated between the hospital in the north of England where her mother was and the antenatal clinic on the south coast that she was attending. There were long journeys in hot or draughty trains. 'I was frightened for the baby because I was under such stress and got so tired. I thought it must be harming the baby. My mother needed me and the baby needed me and Simon needed me. I felt used up.' She says she was enormously surprised when the baby was born perfect: 'She was gorgeous, every hair and finger nail of her.' Felicity breastfed and it all worked well for the first six weeks. But her mother's terminal illness coincided with the feeding crisis that often occurs around six weeks, when many babies suddenly need much more food and the milk supply cannot catch up with demand.

Felicity and Simon dashed north and he took over looking after the baby while Felicity spent as much time as she could with her mother. The baby cried and Simon gave her a bottle. Felicity said it felt like utter failure. After her mother's death she decided to re-stimulate her milk supply by putting the baby to the breast every two hours during the day and kept this up for two days. 'The milk miraculously reappeared.' She is still breastfeeding at ten months. But she makes the point, made by many older women, that she not only misses her mother, but misses her on behalf of her little daughter. She says she is actually thinking now of 'adopting' a granny and is looking around for a suitable candidate!

Some women feel torn between wanting to care for a sick parent and the child's needs and find it a great strain. Several women, however, told me how a grandmother who was ill, or who had lost interest in life, gained a new sparkle with the birth. Some of these grandmothers had recently lost their husbands and were still grieving painfully. A baby helped them to come out of a sometimes prolonged mourning and had enormous psychological benefits.

Having a baby over 35 poses different challenges from having one in your early twenties. But older parents bring experience of life that helps them cope. One said:

I know you can't win every time. When I was 20 I wanted to succeed with everything and I was upset if I didn't. Now I know you are good at some things, and not at others. I reckon I can relax more with a baby than I ever could when I was 20. There are umpteen different ways of doing things and no one best way. I break all the rules about what you are supposed to do and not do, but I enjoy her.

That lesson does not happen with most of us until we have a second baby. The 'how to' books go to the back of the shelf and we get on with discovering the unique personality of that particular child and tackling problems as they come. Older mothers start off with the experience that enables them to enjoy a *first* baby in the same spirit of adventure.

A woman most appreciates a mother who lives near enough to offer regular practical help, rather than advice. As one says: 'She has the baby for an hour at a time and allows me to recharge my batteries.' It is sometimes possible to make friends with an older person in the neighbourhood you can trust who can learn your ways and take over occasionally. An adopted grandmother or father provides a child with another loving adult and the relationship brings pleasure to an otherwise lonely older person.

Some grandmothers see the baby as a threat, depriving them of love. The new mother then feels an extra drain on her strength as she tries to cope with the emotional demands of a lonely and unhappy parent as well as the stresses of dealing with a family, new baby and running a home. She may become very resentful of this parent, whether it is her own or her partner's mother, and it is important that the couple discuss their feelings together and develop a joint strategy to cope with the problem.

Mothers

The birth of a child can profoundly affect the relationship of a woman with her own mother. This change may start in pregnancy. One woman, four months' pregnant, says: 'My parents have, at last, realized that I'm "grown up" now and think twice before telling me what to do.' Some remain in an almost adolescent relationship with their mothers until they have their first baby. If this is not till a woman is over 35, the bond between mother and daughter may have become hard-set, with the older woman treating her daughter as irresponsible, incompetent and in need of protection, and the younger woman being in a continual state of revolt.

But part of the sense of freedom and of having matured that many women experience is that the relationship with their own mothers undergoes rapid change:

We always had a terribly thorny relationship. All of a sudden I've become acceptable. I'm a mother – like her. At the same time, I understand the pressures she has been under as the mother of seven children.

However concerned the older woman is that her daughter cannot look after a baby properly, and even if she offers unwelcome advice in the first few months, after a while the older woman usually begins to realize that her daughter *can* manage. One woman said that finally recovering the happy relationship with her own mother, which came with surrendering her defensiveness and learning to give love, brought deep satisfaction: 'I am sure I was arrogant and selfish before. Loving a little baby is the completest joy.'

Where a woman already has a good relationship with her mother, the sharing between the two women further enriches it. Di said the fact that her mother had successfully breastfed her own four children helped her to develop her own confidence in breastfeeding. Her mother came to stay for a few weeks:

We've always been close but for the first time I really understood the mother/child relationship. She never criticized anything I did, was interested in new ways of doing things, and was able to take my outbursts of temper (mainly due to tiredness) completely in her stride. She was my safety valve.

Where sisters are emotionally close and non-competitive they can give very good postnatal support. It is best not to have to get to know new people when you are most in need of an understanding friend to listen and give relaxed counselling and not be judgemental. Connie, whose two sisters gave her a great deal of support over the telephone, added that she also had a marvellous cleaner and a freezer full of cooked foods. These practical aspects of life can loom large after a baby comes. Some women, though they have sisters who have had babies, cannot happily use them to help during this period because they are still competing with them. Sometimes one element in actually having the baby is that a woman is locked in competition with a sister and wants to prove to her mother or father that she can do as well.

For most women a mother-in-law, even a very understanding one, is classed as a 'visitor' compared with her own mother. On the other hand, the birth of the baby may bring a new mother and mother-in-law closer together. As one woman put it, 'Because I was an academic she didn't know how to treat me. I was "different". Now I've become "normal".' One woman of 36 said:

Since the birth, my relationship with my mother-in-law has improved enormously. I did not feel any particular affinity with her for a long time, and she herself was probably thinking that I might not be good enough for *her son*! When she saw how well I was coping with the pregnancy, she already considered me better, but it was really on the day of the birth that the sudden change occurred. She was delighted with the baby, and in fact I think she was proud of me as well, as I did so well with the birth. And as her son thanked her for her giving birth to him as a baby ('Now I realize what you did!') she really blossomed into an even brighter smile, and her eyes were shining with the joy of being recognized, maybe for the first time in her life, and that by her son!

Sometimes a new mother knows already that she cannot cope with her mother-in-law for more than short periods at a time and that these have to be carefully planned in advance. If this is so, it is vital to discuss it with your partner so that he knows the strategy, realizes that you need his protection, and is not left feeling disloyal to both women. Connie, who got on well with her own mother, was usually great friends with her husband's mother too. But the two could not agree about Connie's style of breastfeeding and she knew that her mother-in-law was worried about prolonged breastfeeding and Dan getting interrupted sleep at nights. The baby was breastfed whenever she wanted until she was 16 months. At 15 months she had a throat infection and rejected other foods, having 14 feeds a day, not including those at night. 'I know,' said Connie, 'because my mother-in-law whom we were staying with and who was disgusted with the whole thing had counted for me!' Once the infection cleared up she weaned herself in four days. 'That was one-in-the-eye for my mother-in-law, who is actually normally a very understanding person.'

This is a bonus of breastfeeding. It is the perfect food if the child is ill, and may not only be the most comforting one, but the only one she can digest and wants. In my own experience most crises in breast-feeding, when women seek help urgently, together with anxiety about not yet having weaned a child, come at times of the year when there are family gatherings and members of the family go to stay with one another, such as Christmas and Easter or the summer holidays.

In some ways the older mother is immunized from the criticisms of those to whom she is nearest by her own experience of life. She knows that there is more than one way of doing things and that they probably all work. She is, as one woman put it, 'less of a perfectionist and more of a human being', and is better able to relax and enjoy her baby than she would have been in her twenties.

9

Coping alone

A woman alone faces special challenges in pregnancy if only because she feels the whole burden of responsibility for planning ahead, supporting the child financially, and loving, rests on her shoulders. If she is over 35 she tends to take this on with understanding, born from her experience of life, more than a woman still in her teens or twenties.

For some women deciding to have a baby when they are in their thirties, the child is their 'last chance', and conception is the consequence of a carefully thought-out decision. Some cannot find the right man and are concerned only to have a child. Some do not wish to be with a man anyway and prefer a loving relationship with another woman. A lesbian mother is usually not alone, and the relationship with her partner is often a good deal more stable than many heterosexual relationships. The woman who chooses self-insemination has also taken time to work out what she wants and conception is far from the accident that it often is in a male–female partnership.

Other women are having a child after separating from the baby's father, and occasionally after his death. The woman alone is, therefore, not 'one person' but many – and these various 'sub-groups' may in fact have little in common with one another.

A woman with no partner needs a good support network both before and after the baby is born. To start with, it is vital that she has a companion who goes with her to classes, works with her on breathing and relaxation, and understands exactly how to help in labour. To plan on having someone at the birth simply to hold your hand is not enough. You need someone to really share the labour and who has the skills to help you keep on an even course. This can be a woman friend, sister or other relative, antenatal teacher (or one who is studying to be one), and I have known women who have had a trusted man friend take this on too. A charming and sophisticated older man attended every single class in one course – on time even when his friend was late – accepting the responsibility because the father of her child was in his late teens and could not face it. This older man was present throughout labour and delivery, experienced the rush of emotions that a new father usually does, and then had to stand back as the younger biological father decided that he liked the idea of being a dad after all, now that the baby had arrived safely.

Birth companions

One woman selected two lovers as birth companions. They were, according to the midwife, both 'marvellous', and, she added, 'I'm not sure which I would have chosen!' Another woman spent the major part of the first stage of labour with friends who lived near the hospital, a couple whom she had got to know in the childbirth class, and whose own baby was three weeks old. The father of this baby had support techniques fresh in his mind, had learned from his wife's experience, and shepherded her through with sensitivity and skill.

The important thing is that the single woman has someone with her whose task it is to concentrate on her needs as a *person*, not a reproductive body, and whose responsibilities are not divided between his relationship and medical tasks. This is why it is not enough to rely on a midwife for this, however kind and caring she is.

In some hospitals, even today a woman may find herself left alone in labour. When wards are full, drugs may be used by busy members of staff in place of personal help and understanding. Pat says she went into hospital far too early, probably because she was alone and felt she could not cope by herself if she left it till the contractions were coming five minutes apart:

> The contractions stopped for about twelve hours, but it was nice because they weren't busy and the nurses all talked about how I was going to manage on my own and seemed genuinely interested. Unfortunately, Andrew decided to be born at their busy time and the entirely unsympathetic night staff had taken over. I was totally out of control, couldn't do any of the exercises I'd practised so assiduously, and felt a complete coward. In the end, they gave me an injection and put me out.

An alternative arrangement is for this companion – a *doula* – to be with you at home so that you can spend early labour in familiar surroundings, rather than only turning up at the hospital. It helps to get into the rhythm of breathing and relaxing in the first half of the first stage in a close partnership, without the intrusion of other people if this can be avoided. Susan, whose lover was abroad and whom she did not want to involve any more than he wished, because she had not consulted him about starting the pregnancy, says that no one can ever talk to her of independence who has not made the journey alone to hospital to have a baby and then, days later, come out of it, going to the car park, collecting the baby at the maternity entrance, and driving off.

A doula should have the knowledge to be able to be a 'patient advocate' if necessary. A woman in labour needs to be able to rely on someone to say if she is in the middle of a contraction and does not wish to have an injection of pethidine, to remind her that she should be given a vaginal examination immediately before having an epidural just in case she is already almost fully dilated, or perhaps to say, before an episiotomy (a surgical cut to enlarge the birth opening) is done, that her friend in labour did hope she might be able to manage without one and would it be possible to see if 'breathing the baby out' would help. A patient advocate cannot, by definition, be an employee of the hospital. Anybody working for the hospital is bound to have divided loyalties. To say this may be hurtful to a midwife who sees her role as being on her patient's side, but, as Norma Swenson[1] of the Boston Women's Health Group points out, though attractive as a concept, an alliance between consumers and professionals is unrealistic because a woman having a baby has transient and unequal status in the hospital system.

Often a doula can attend at least some of the clinics too and look round the hospital in advance. A birth companion unfamiliar with hospitals may find this especially helpful. One woman, reluctant about getting fully involved with her partner's birth, felt much more relaxed about this after meeting friendly staff. She said she now began to see her role more clearly and would not feel out of place.

Powerful emotions

With other partners, just as with husbands, strong emotions are often involved, and it is a mistake to think that a companion is there simply to remind you of exercises or rub your back. One man, married with two small children, who had been present at the births of both of them, supported his mistress through a pregnancy with his child, doing so because he felt it was right, though he was unwilling to break up his marriage. Duty, responsibility, compassion, whatever he felt, gave way to passionate outpouring of emotion as he relived the births of his other children. He expressed his pain and joy, and in some inexplicable way this assurance of his emotional surrender to the experience gave the woman who was bearing his child great psychological support.

Another, attending classes with her lesbian partner, had herself had a pregnancy the previous year that had finished in a late miscarriage. It must have been stressful for her to allow herself to identify with the woman having the baby and give herself completely to her in loving support, but she did.

Sometimes the choice of support partner is a woman's own mother. It is vitally important for the mother to share preparation with her daughter if she is to be with her in labour. Not only have birth styles changed, with apparatus that the mother may not have seen before, but women tend to bring their own experiences of childbearing with them into the birth they attend. If these were unhappy, a mother may not be able to help her daughter to feel confident.

Faith's mother was deeply distressed to learn that her unmarried daughter was pregnant. She prayed that she be saved from sin every day. She did not know what to do, whether to turn Faith away or look forward to the birth of the baby with her. She spoke to the pastor at the Evangelical church she attended, who suggested that the right thing was to give her daughter her unconditional love. Faith was very happy with her mother's changed attitude and, at my suggestion, asked her if she would come to childbirth classes with her. Faith said she had always been very inhibited about anything to do with sex and did not know how her mother would take all the talk about bodies and feelings. Her own labour had been a terrible and frightening ordeal for her mother. Faith's mother had never had another baby because of what she had suffered while giving birth to Faith. In the event, Faith need not have worried. Her mother, brought up in ignorance of her body, was hungry for information and obviously enjoyed the group, asked many questions, discussed vigorously with other couples present, and told me that her life would have been so different if she had known all this earlier and been able to see it for the miracle it was. She supported her daughter magnificently through a drug-free labour and the two became friends as never before.

The role of the support person can, perhaps, be best illustrated by describing the way a particular partnership worked during a painful, induced labour in which a Caesarean section was always on the cards and a forceps delivery very likely. The support that this single mother had from another woman gave her the confidence, courage and trust in her body that resulted in a spontaneous birth.

Felicity had been warned that she would probably need a Caesarean section. She was having a big baby and was of small build. Joanna, her friend, had a baby daughter herself. She came to classes with Felicity, determined to give her full support through what was an emotionally difficult time, not only because of the uncertainty about the birth, but because Felicity was beginning to realize that the father of her baby was not going to leave his wife and children, and was very anxious that it might leak out that he had fathered a baby outside the marriage. Both women kept careful notes during as much of the labour as they could and wrote the rest up immediately afterwards, as you can see from Joanna's diary extract that follows.

Joanna's diary

Joanna's diary starts when the midwife rang from the hospital to say that the induction had started and Felicity was asking for her:

'Packed ice into thermos and shot off in taxi. Did relaxing exercises myself in taxi so would bring a calm reassuring atmosphere with me.'

Once there, the first thing Joanna had to do was to work out the best place to stand in the room, which was equipped spaceship style. She needed to be out of the midwife's way, not obstructing the equipment, yet close enough to Felicity to touch and hold her when she seemed to want this. She could see from the clock that each contraction was lasting about 45 seconds:

'. . . but felt the best thing for me to do was to watch Felicity and try to see what she wanted. I talked to her between contractions, making her laugh a bit because I felt that was what she needed, and keeping silent with just my hand on her arm during contractions, watching her face and hands and feet to see if they were tensing up, and occasionally just lightly stroking her shoulder for reassurance and to check that it was relaxed. In between contractions I checked that the thermos with ice was to hand and cloths and lip salve.'

'I made a point of asking everyone who came in for any length of time what their name was, as I felt that the more personal the process was, the more confident Felicity would be, and once somebody has given you their name there is less tendency to be high-handed.'

After about one and a half hours contractions were stronger:

'. . . and from now on I didn't move away from her at all . . . If I moved from one side to let the midwives get at the equipment I moved to the other or held her feet very gently until I could put my hand on her upper arm, which was where she seemed to prefer it.'

'The machine monitoring the contractions and the baby's heartbeat was not functioning too well, so there was quite a lot of coming and going and tinkering about, which Felicity found distracting. So every time it happened I told her quietly not to take any notice of them, they weren't important (which must have gone down a treat if they heard).'

Somebody came to deal with the monitor. Joanna asked him firmly but politely to keep his voice down:

'He seemed surprised and obviously thought it rather funny. Then a staff nurse told Felicity to turn over and started to move her mid-contraction. I said, quietly, so as not to disturb Felicity, "Could you wait until this contraction is over?" She said, "But she has to turn on her side." I said, "Yes, but not now. Could it wait a minute? Then she could help you herself." It must have carried force because although she looked daggers she waited until I said, "OK", and then we got Felicity over and tried to make her as comfy as possible.'

After another two and a quarter hours, Felicity said she could not bear any more and she would like pethidine, but immediately she had the injection she started to feel desperate and said she wanted an epidural:

'I told her the pethidine took a quarter of an hour to work, that although it must seem like for ever, did she want to try and ride out the quarter of an hour? I promised I would tell her when it was up. I said that if she didn't want to wait I'd get someone to do the epidural. She said she would wait, and between contractions I told her the time and how much longer there was to go till the end of the quarter of an hour. I could see the pethidine had started to work and I told her, and when she said that she was OK, told her how well she was doing and how wonderfully she had got through the quarter of an hour.'

Felicity says:

'I coped only with Jo. Without her I might have gone under.'

This is how Felicity describes the help that Joanna gave her:

'She was encouraging me all the time, saying "Relax into it – you're doing very well – very good", and praising and encouraging me. Throughout, a battery of doctors and nurses kept coming in and the monitoring equipment kept going wrong.'

The clip on the baby's head was not registering the foetal heart, so another monitor was strapped round her abdomen:

'After five hours I was beginning to tire of riding the pain. Jo said, "Don't worry about the other people, just breathe, keep breathing, you're doing well, you've made it, well done!". . . At the point where I was tired a midwife did a VE and I was only five to six centimetres dilated! I thought another five hours of this is impossible, but Jo said to me, "You know it goes much quicker from now on." '

Felicity said it was 'a marathon'. She kept asking Joanna for water, who put a small sponge soaked in icy water from the thermos in her mouth to suck. Her mouth became very dry because when she reached the end of the first stage most of her breathing was done through it. Sometimes Joanna could hardly get to the flask before another contraction came:

'She also wiped my face with a warm cloth. I especially liked to feel that on my cheeks and her warm hand on my arm through the contractions.'

At last she began to want to push and Joanna takes over the story again:

'I kept gently tipping her head down so that her chin was tucked in as she tended to throw her head back. There seemed to be no progress and the doctor came in ready to do a forceps delivery. Then as they got her feet into the stirrups the baby's head rounded the corner and Felicity said she could feel it. Someone looked and said, "I can see the top of the head." I said to Felicity, "You're going to do it yourself after all." The doctor said, "I think I'm going to see a normal birth. I haven't seen one for years. See if you can break my run." I dashed down to see and saw a little dark mass and rushed up and told her I could see the baby's head.'

Felicity pushed, the baby slid out, and was given to her to hold immediately. Black tendrils of hair damp from the womb, cheeks like a ripe peach, and huge eyes, violet-blue, looking straight up at her. She was plump and firm and amazingly hot, straight from a tropical uterine climate. Felicity was laughing and crying at the same time. She drew the baby closer, holding her hungrily, devouring with her eyes the reality of this little person who stared at her quite calmly as if to say: 'So, this is my mother!' Joanna was crying too. Her arm was round Felicity as she held the child.

A chance to grow

Birth can be, and is for many women, an opening up of the new, an unfolding of love, not only for the baby, but for those from whom we have been guarding and protecting ourselves, and a step on the journey towards deeper understanding of ourselves and others. We can never possess our children. But, through them, and with their help, we have a chance to grow as human beings.

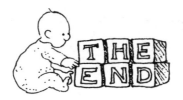

Notes

Introduction

1 Office of National Statistics, HMSO, London, 2009.
2 Kitzinger, S., *The New Pregnancy and Childbirth: Choices and Challenges*, Dorling Kindersley, London, 2008.
3 Kitzinger, S., *The New Experience of Childbirth*, Orion, London, 2004.
4 Kitzinger, S., *Birth Your Way*, Fresh Heart, Chester le Street, 2011.

1 Deciding to have a baby

1 Office of National Statistics, HMSO, London, 2009.

2 Planning ahead for pregnancy

1 Wilkins, L., 'Masculinization of the female foetus due to use of orally given progesterone', *Journal of American Medical Association*, 1960; 172: 1028–32.
2 Harlap, S. *et al.*, 'Birth defects and oestrogen and progesterone in pregnancy', *Lancet*, 1975: 692–3.
3 Seigal, D. and Corfman, P., 'Epidemiological problems associated with studies of the safety of oral contraceptives', *Journal of American Medical Association*, 1968; 203: 950.
4 Robertson-Rintoul, J., 'Oral contraception: potential hazards of hormone therapy during pregnancy', *Lancet*, 1974: 1315.
5 Seaman B. and Seaman G., *Women and the Crisis in Sex Hormones*, Bantam, New York, 1978.
6 Bernard, R., 'Factors governing IUD performance', *American Journal of Public Health*, 1971; 61: 559–6.
7 Smithells, R. *et al.*, 'Possible prevention of neural-tube defects by pre-conceptual vitamin supplement', *Lancet*, 1980: 339–40.
8 Laurence, K. *et al.*, 'Double-blind randomized controlled trial of folate treatment before conception to prevent recurrence of neural-tube defects', *British Medical Journal*, 1981; 282: 1509–11.
9 Hofmejr, G. *et al.*, 'Calcium supplementation during pregnancy for preventing hypertensive disorder and related problems', *Cochrane Database of Systematic Reviews*, issue 8, 2010.
10 Pirani, B., 'Smoking during pregnancy', *Obstetrics and Gynecology Survey*, 1978; 33:1: 1–13.
11 US Department of Health, Education and Welfare, *Smoking and Health, A Report of the Surgeon General*, 1979, chapter 8.

12 'Cigarette smoking in pregnancy', editorial in *British Medical Journal*, 28 August 1976 2(6034): 492.
13 'The foetal alcohol syndrome', *Drug Abuse and Alcoholism Newsletter II*, 4 May 1978.
14 Stirrat, G. and McIntyre, G., Adapted from *Obstetrics*, London, 1981.
15 Woodward, S., 'How does strenuous maternal exercise affect the foetus?', *Birth and the Family Journal*, 1981: 8:1.
16 Miller, P. *et al.*, 'Maternal hyperthermia as a possible cause of anencephaly', *Lancet*, 1978; 8063: 519–21.

3 Will the baby be all right?

1 Keatinge, R. and Williams, E., 'Prenatal screening for Down's syndrome', *British Medical Journal*, 1991; 303: 54–5.
2 Varley, W., 'Miracles in the womb', *Parents*, April 1989: 56–9.
3 Taylor, C., 'Ignorance meant we nearly lost Harry', *Independent*, 17 December 1991.
4 Hook, E. and Cross, D., 'Estimated rates of clinically significant cytogenetic abnormality (other than Down's syndrome) by one-year maternal age intervals', *American Journal of Human Genetics*, 1979; 31: 136a.
5 Personal communication with Kypros Nicolaides, Director of Harris Centre for Foetal Research, Kings College Hospital, London.
6 Bucher, J. and Schmidt, J., 'Does routine ultrasound scanning improve outcome in pregnancy? Meta-analysis of various outcome measures', *British Medical Journal*, 1981; 307: 13–17; Saari-Kemppainen, A. *et al.*, 'Helsinki Ultrasound Trial', *Lancet*, 1990; 336: 387–91.
7 Marles, K., 'I felt like I was killing my baby . . . while my instincts were to protect it', *Good Housekeeping*, September 1990.
8 Statham, H. and Green, J., 'Serum screening for Down's syndrome: some women's experiences', *British Medical Journal*, 1993; 307: 174–6.
9 Green, J. *et al.*, 'Screening for foetal abnormalities: attitudes and experiences', in Chard, T. and Richards, M., eds, *Obstetrics in the 1990s: Current Controversies. Clinics in Developmental Medicine 123/124*, MacKeith Press, London, 1992.
10 Marles, 'I felt like I was killing my baby'.
11 Meade, T. and Grant, A., 'Chorionic villus sampling', *British Medical Journal*, 1992; 304: 185–6.
12 Statham and Green, 'Serum screening for Down's syndrome'.
13 Weiner, C., 'Use of cordocentesis in foetal haemolytic disease and auto-immune thrombocytopenia', *American Journal of Obstetrics and Gynecology*, 1990; 162: 1126–7.
14 SATFA. http//www.arc-uk.org.
15 Statham, H., 'Professional understanding and parents' experience of termination', in Brock, K. *et al.*, *Perinatal Diagnosis and Screening*, Churchill Livingstone, London, 1992.

16 Love, E. R., Bhattacharya, S., Smith, N. C. *et al.*, 'Effect of interpregnancy interval on outcomes of pregnancy after miscarriage: retrospective analysis of hospital episode statistics in Scotland', *British Medical Journal*, 2010; 341: c3967.

4 The clinic

1 'Dietary interventions and physical activity interventions for weight management before, during and after pregnancy', NICE, 2010.
2 Hertogs, K. *et al.*, 'Maternal perception of foetal motoractivity', *British Medical Journal*, 1979; 6199: 1183–5.
3 Pearson, J. and Weaver, J., 'Foetal activity and foetal wellbeing', *British Medical Journal*, 1976; 1(6021): 1305–7.
4 Pearson, J., 'Foetal movements', *Nursing Mirror*, 21 April 1977.
5 Rayburn, W. *et al.*, 'Maternal perception of foetal movement and perinatal outcome', *Obstetrics and Gynecology*, 1980; 56:2: 161–5.
6 Lewis, A., *An Interesting Condition: The Diary of a Pregnant Woman*, Odhams, London, 1951.
7 Roberts, A. *et al.*, '24 hour studies of foetal respiratory movements and foetal body movements in normal and abnormal pregnancies', *The Current Status of Foetal Heart Rate Monitoring and Ultrasound in Obstetrics*, RCOG, London, 1977: 209–20.

5 Doctors

1 Laurance, J., 'One in five hospital trusts found to be putting mothers and babies at risk: How good is your maternity hospital?' *Independent*, 25 January 2008.
2 NICE, Healthcare Commission, 2007.
3 Chalmers, I., 'Confronting therapeutic ignorance', *British Medical Journal*, 2008; 337: 246–7.
4 Scully, D., *Men Who Control Women's Health*, Houghton Mifflin, Boston, 1980.
5 Oakley, A., *Subject Women*, Robertson, Oxford, 1981.
6 Byrne, P. and Long, P., *Doctors Talking to Patients*, HMSO, London, 1976.
7 Chalmers, I., Enkin, M. and Keirse, M. (eds), *Effective Care in Pregnancy and Childbirth*, Oxford University Press, 1989.
8 Francis, H., 'Obstetrics: a consumer oriented service? The case against', *Maternal and Child Health*, 1985; 10:3: 69.
9 'Late-bloomers: giving birth after 35', *Birth Gazette*, 1986; 3:1: 16–17.
10 Downe, S. and Dykes, F., 'Counting time in pregnancy and labour', in McCourt, C. (ed.), *Childbirth, Midwifery and Concepts of Time*, Berghahn Books, New York, 2010.
11 Kitzinger, S., *Some Women's Experiences of Induction*, National Childbirth Trust, London, 2nd edn 1978.

12 Klaus, M. and Kennell, J., *Maternal-infant Bonding*, Mosby, St Louis, 1976.
13 Donald, I., *Practical Obstetric Problems*, Lloyd-Luke, London, 1979.
14 'The changing epidemiology of mortality and morbidity in mothers and babies in recent years'. Paper presented at a study group on problems in obstetrics organized by the Medical Information Unit of the Spastics Society, Tunbridge Wells, April 1975.
15 Tipton, R. and Lewis, B., 'Induction of labour and perinatal mortality', *British Medical Journal*, 1975; 1(5954): 391.
16 'Induction and the acceleration of labour in modern obstetric practice'. Paper presented at a study group on problems in obstetrics organized by the Medical Information Unit of the Spastics Society, Tunbridge Wells, April 1975.
17 Donald, *Practical Obstetric Problems*.
18 Lumley, J. and Astbury, J., *Birth Rites, Birth Rights*, Sphere, Australia, 1980.
19 Cahill, A. *et al.*, 'Vaginal birth after caesarean for women with three or more prior caesareans: assessing safety and success', *British Journal of Obstetrics and Gynaecology*, 2010; 117(4): 422–8.
20 Lumley and Astbury, *Birth Rites, Birth Rights*.
21 Mitchell, R., 'Antecedents of handicap', *Lancet*, 1981; 821: 86–7.

6 Life after the baby comes

1 Permission to reproduce sought.
2 Atwood, M., *The Edible Woman*, Virago, London, 1980.
3 Klaus, M. H. and Kennell, J. H., *Maternal Infant Bonding*, Mosby, St Louis, 1976.
4 'Helping mothers to love their babies', *British Medical Journal*, 1977; 2(6087): 595–6.
5 National Childbirth Trust Breastfeeding Helpline 0300 330 0771, <www.nctpregnancyandbabycare.com>.

7 Partners

1 Bowlby, J., *Maternal Care and Mental Health*, World Health Organisation, 1951; Bowlby, J., *Childcare and the Growth of Love*, Penguin, 1953; Bowlby, J., *Attachment*, Penguin, 1971.
2 Schaffer, J. and Emerson, P., 'The development of social attachments in infancy', *Monographs of Social Research in Child Development*, 1964; 29:3: 1–77.
3 Bourguignon, E., *A World of Women*, Praeger, New York, 1980.
4 Lannoy, R., *The Speaking Tree: A Study of Indian Culture and Society*, Oxford University Press, 1971.
5 Kitzinger, S., unpublished research in Jamaica.
6 Kitzinger, S., *Ourselves as Mothers*, Bantam, London, 1993.

7 Porter, A., 'Depressive illness in general practice', *British Medical Journal*, 1970; 1(5699): 773–8.
8 Bardwick J. *et al.*, *Feminine Personality and Conflict*, Wadsworth, California, 1970.
9 Oakley, A., *Subject Women*, Robertson, Oxford, 1981.
10 Klaus, M. and Kennell, J., *Maternal-infant Bonding*, Mosby, St Louis, 1976.

9 Coping alone

1 *Maternity Care in Ferment*, Maternity Center Association, New York, 1980.

Index